D94

Treatment of MIGRAINE

Treatment of MIGRAINE

Pharmacological & Biofeedback Considerations

Edited by
Roy J. Mathew, M.D., D.P.M., M.R.C. Psych.
Chief, Psychosomatic Research Section
Texas Research Institute of Mental Sciences
Houston

Technical Editors
Lore Feldman
Karen Hanson Stuyck

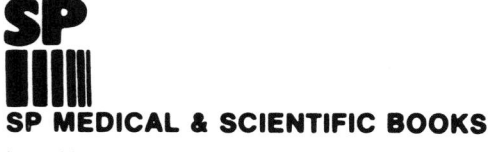

SP MEDICAL & SCIENTIFIC BOOKS
New York

Proceedings of Symposium, November 30–December 1, 1979, sponsored by the Texas Research Institute of Mental Sciences, Houston

Copyright © 1981 Spectrum Publications

All rights reserved. No part of this book may be reproduced in any form, by photostat, microform, retrieval system, or any other means without prior written permission of the copyright holder or his licensee.

SPECTRUM PUBLICATIONS, INC.
175-20 Wexford Terrace, Jamaica, N.Y. 11432

Library of Congress Cataloging in Publication Data
Main entry under title:

Treatment of migraine.

   Includes bibliographies and index.
   Contents: Measurements of regional cerebral blood flow (rCBF) and their application to migraine research / John Stirling Meyer — Complicated migraine and differential diagnosis of migraine / Ninan T. Mathew — Pharmacological treatment of migraine / Seymour Diamond and Jose L. Medina — [etc.]
   1. Migraine. 2. Migraine—Chemotherapy. 3. Biofeedback training. 4. Analgesics. I. Mathew, Roy J. [DNLM: 1. Biofeedback (Psychology) 2. Migraine—Drug therapy. 3. Migraine—Therapy. WL 344 T784]
RC392.T73   616.8′5706   81-8937
ISBN 0-89335-148-2   AACR2

Contributors

TIM A. AHLES, B.A.
Department of Psychology
State University of New York at Albany
Albany, New York

EDWARD B. BLANCHARD, Ph.D.
Department of Psychology
State University of New York at Albany
Albany, New York

JAMES L. CLAGHORN, M.D.
Texas Research Institute of Mental
 Sciences
 and
Department of Psychiatry
University of Texas Medical School at
 Houston
 and
Department of Psychiatry
Baylor College of Medicine
Houston, Texas

SEYMOUR DIAMOND, M.D.
Diamond Headache Clinic
 and
Department of Neurology
Chicago Medical School
Chicago, Illinois

JUDI DIAMOND-FALK
Diamond Headache Clinic
Chicago, Illinois

BENG T. HO, Ph.D.
Neurochemistry and Neuropharmacology
 Research Section
Texas Research Institute of Mental
 Sciences
 and
Department of Mental Sciences and
 Pharmacology
University of Texas Health Science
 Center at Houston
Houston, Texas

LEE KUDROW, M.D.
Director, California Medical Clinic for
 Headache
Encino, California

JOHN W. LARGEN, JR., Ph.D.
Neuropsychology Research Section
Texas Research Institute of Mental
 Sciences
Houston, Texas

NINAN T. MATHEW, M.D.
Houston Headache Clinic
 and
Department of Neurology
University of Texas Medical School at
 Houston
Houston, Texas

ROY J. MATHEW, M.D., D.P.M.,
M.R.C. Psych.
Psychosomatic Research Section
Texas Research Institute of Mental
  Sciences
  and
University of Texas Medical School at
  Houston
Houston, Texas

JOSE L. MEDINA, M.D.
Diamond Headache Clinic
  and
Department of Neurology
Chicago Medical School
Chicago, Illinois

JOHN STIRLING MEYER, M.D.
Department of Neurology
Baylor College of Medicine
  and
Regional Cerebral Blood Flow Laboratory
Veterans Administration Medical Center
Houston, Texas

JOSEPH D. SARGENT, M.D.
Department of Internal Medicine
  and
Headache Research and Treatment
  Project
The Menninger Foundation
Topeka, Kansas

MAXINE L. WEINMAN, D.P.H.
Psychosomatic Research Section
Texas Research Institute of Mental
  Sciences
  and
University of Texas School of Public
  Health
Houston, Texas

Contents

   Introduction
      Roy J. Mathew

1 Measurements of Regional Cerebral Blood Flow (rCBF) and Their Application to Migraine Research   1
      John Stirling Meyer

2 Complicated Migraine and Differential Diagnosis of Migraine   9
      Ninan T. Mathew

3 Pharmacological Treatment of Migraine   27
      Seymour Diamond and Jose L. Medina

4 Update: Biofeedback in the Treatment of Vascular Headache   37
      Seymour Diamond, Judi Diamond-Falk, and John W. Largen, Jr.

5 Biochemistry of Migraine   67
      Lee Kudrow

6 Integration of Psychosomatic Self-Regulation of Headache into Medically Recognized Therapies   77
      Joseph D. Sargent

7 Cerebral Blood Flow and Headache Activity in Normal Volunteers and Migraineurs Trained in Skin Temperature Self-Regulation   91
      John W. Largen, Jr., and Roy J. Mathew

8 Biochemistry of Biofeedback Treatment   127
      Roy J. Mathew and Beng T. Ho

9 Evaluation of Relaxation Training as Treatment for Migraine Headaches   141
      Edward B. Blanchard and Tim A. Ahles

10 A Study of Physicians' Attitudes on Biofeedback   153
      Maxine L. Weinman, Roy J. Mathew, and James L. Claghorn

   Index   167

Introduction

Biofeedback has brought forth two important concepts: the possibility of volitional control over involuntary body functions and nonpharmacological treatment of some physical illnesses. Both concepts are appealing to patients as well as to therapists. In a society that deems self-sufficiency an important virtue, the possibility of conscious control over physical functions seems highly desirable. For chronically ill patients who must rely on drugs indefinitely despite the known and unknown side effects, liberation from the pill bottle would be the ultimate hope; the enthusiasm with which biofeedback was received by the public is understandable.

The advent of this new nonpharmacological form of treatment, however, and its immediate popularity have given rise to several controversies. Many clinicians believe that the first flush of enthusiasm for biofeedback led to widespread clinical application of the technique before its indications and contraindications were adequately investigated. Biofeedback clinics have sprouted all over the country; people from widely differing backgrounds—physicians, psychologists, nurses, social workers, pastoral counselors, and some unqualified persons—have entered the field. The distrust some clinicians felt about premature clinical application of biofeedback was sharpened by the presence of charlatan therapists.

The resultant heated controversies and confusion have, to some extent, overshadowed issues related to biofeedback, which are of considerable scientific and practical significance. An impressive volume of scientific research reports has accumulated which supports the therapeutic value of biofeedback for certain well-defined illnesses. Migraine is one of these. Although the American Society for the Study of Headache has endorsed biofeedback as a valid therapy for migraine, the controversy that surrounds biofeedback as a whole touches biofeedback treatment of headaches as well. Many physicians who treat patients for headache seem to be unaware of the scientific basis of this behavioral technique. Conversely, many nonphysicians who treat migraine patients with behavioral techniques seem to be unfamiliar with the medical aspects of the illness. Obviously, knowledge of both the pharmacological and behavioral aspects of the illness would enable clinicians to offer patients a treatment plan best suited to their needs. Such understanding would be valuable to the researcher and the clinician, and would serve as an additional vista to the pathology of migraine headaches.

This book is meant for physicians and nonphysicians who treat patients with migraine headaches. It provides information about the diagnosis of migraine, its etiology, course, complications, and pharmacological treatment. The application of biofeedback in treating this illness is examined in detail. Possible physiological and biochemical mechanisms of migraine are discussed. Biofeedback is still young; the information presented in this volume is preliminary, awaiting further replication and substantiation. We hope that this book will add to knowledge of pharmacological and behavioral treatments for migraine, in the service of better therapy for headache patients.

Roy J. Mathew, M.D.

Treatment of MIGRAINE

Chapter 1

Measurements of Regional Cerebral Blood Flow (rCBF) and Their Application to Migraine Research

JOHN STIRLING MEYER, M.D.

METHODS FOR NONINVASIVE rCBF MEASUREMENTS

Regional cerebral blood flow (rCBF), supplying 16 separate regions of both hemispheres, brainstem, and cerebellum, is measured noninvasively by a modification of the ^{133}Xenon (Xe) inhalation method [1], using a bicompartmental algorithm originally programmed for computer analysis by Obrist and colleagues [2]. The method is based on a modification of the Fick principle, using inhalation of the radioisotope ^{133}Xe (which emits gamma and x-rays) as the indicator. Arterial recirculation is corrected by deconvoluting the head curve with the end-tidal ^{133}Xe curve (or PE ^{133}Xe), which is in equilibrium with the arterial blood. The head curves or desaturation of Xe from brain is recorded by collimated sodium iodide crystals, utilizing a computer program of our own design. By these means the computer provides a hard-copy printout including a brain map, showing the regional rCBF values to the left and normal values to the right with standard deviations as determined in this laboratory (Figs. 1A, B). For each region, gray matter flow (Fg), white matter flow (Fw), mean 10-minute flow or flow infinity (F_{10} or F_∞), and weight of gray matter are provided. If the weight of gray matter, normally 45 to 50 percent, is reduced, this is an index of gray matter atrophy.

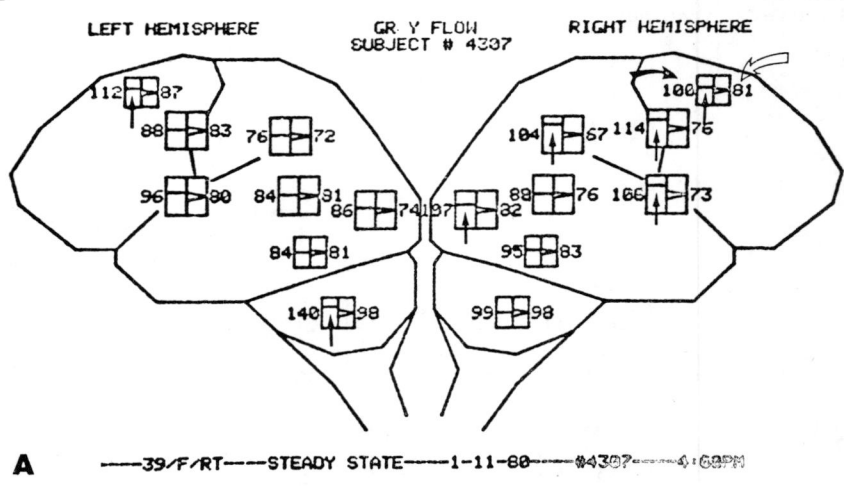

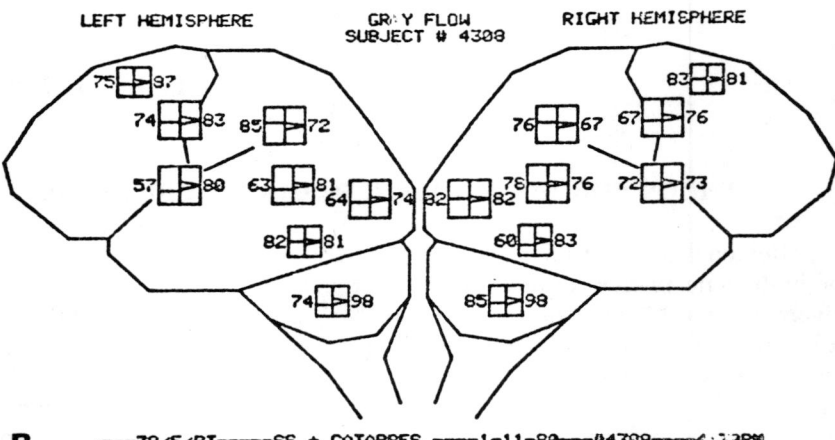

Figure 1. (A) Computer printout of rCBF Fg values in patient with common migraine during onset of typical unilateral headache (marked "steady state"). To right of each box are normal values for age-matched controls, indicated by open curved arrow with standard deviation indicated by >. At left of each box, solid curved arrow indicates patient's values. Vertical solid arrow indicates elevated Fg values typically recorded during headache interval. (B) Shows repeat measurements made one hour after ingestion of 0.2 mg of centrally acting α-blocker clonidine (Catapres) which lowered BP 11 mm Hg. Flow values returned to normal due to impaired autoregulation and headache has subsided.

^{133}Xe is inhaled for one minute through a face mask (Fig. 2A). After this, each rCBF measurement requires a 10-minute desaturation interval, during which time clearance curves from the head are recorded by the computer. The faster the flow, the more rapid the clearance and vice versa. The method is noninvasive, and there have been no ill effects during this laboratory's experience with 6000 successful measurements in hospital patients, outpatients, and normal, healthy volunteers.

The electroencephalograph (EEG), electrocardiograph (EKG), end-tidal ^{133}Xenon (PE ^{133}Xe), end-tidal oxygen (PEO$_2$), body temperature, pulse, respiration, and end-tidal CO$_2$ (PECO$_2$) are recorded concurrently on a polygraph during the rCBF measurements. The collimated probes are mounted in a modified motorcycle helmet (Fig. 2B), which permits simultaneous measurement of the clearance of long penetrating gamma rays from the brain and short penetrating x-rays from the scalp. This makes possible estimation of both scalp and brain blood flow. rCBF measurements are made from the frontal, temporal, parietal, and occipital regions of both hemispheres as well as from the brainstem-cerebellar regions.

APPLICATION TO MIGRAINE RESEARCH

The fact that these rCBF measurements are noninvasive and can be taken on outpatients makes them ideal for clinical research in migraine. Patients can report to the laboratory for rCBF measurements when they have a migraine prodrome, a headache, or are free of headaches, so that comparative serial measurements are possible. Likewise, a cerebral vasodilator challenge induced by inhalation of 5-percent CO$_2$ may be carried out and the pharmacological effects of different medications evaluated (Figure 2A, B). One can also look at the regional distribution of the CBF changes, before and during a migraine attack. Thus, during the headache phase of classical migraine and of Bickerstaff's basilar type of migraine [3] the increase in rCBF usually is located primarily in the territory of the basilar artery. During the prodrome of classical migraine, and in complicated migraine, rCBF values are decreased in the territory corresponding to the patient's neurological complaints. During the prodrome of a classical migraine headache, for example, there is reduced flow in the occipital areas, with regional increase in rCBF in these same areas during the headache phase. In patients with hemisensory impairment as part of their prodrome, hemispheric rCBF is decreased in both parietal regions, but to a more marked degree in the hemisphere contralateral to the sensory loss.

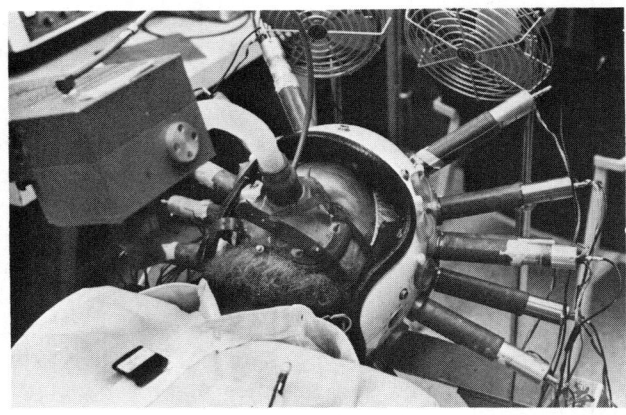
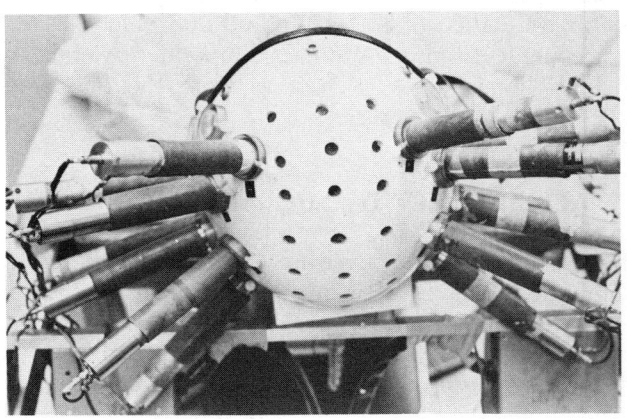

Figure 2. (A) Patient undergoing ^{133}Xe inhalation measurement of regional cerebral blood flow. Helmet is mounted with 16 detector-probes over both hemispheres and brainstem-cerebellar areas. EEG and EKG are recorded, and pulse, temperature, and blood pressure are recorded from finger plethysmograph. Face mask is used for delivery of ^{133}Xe by inhalation and for sampling blood gases from end-tidal air. (B) Rear of helmet showing probes over brainstem and cerebellar regions.

Observations made in this laboratory of patients with classical migraine may be summarized by stating that, during the prodrome, rCBF values are asymmetrically decreased; in the headache interval of classic migraine, common migraine, and cluster headache rCBF values are asymmetrically increased. In the interheadache interval, however, rCBF values are normal for all these types. In contrast, patients with muscle contraction headache show normal rCBF before and during their headaches [4].

Some 20 years ago, Harold G. Wolff, a pioneer of migraine research, postulated that migraine and vascular headaches (such as cluster headache) are caused by unstable neurogenic cerebrovascular control [5]. We tested this theory in patients with vascular headache by measuring rCBF during inhalation of a mixture of 5-percent CO_2 in air, and found it to be correct. Patients with migraine showed excessive cerebral vasodilator responsiveness to 5-percent CO_2 inhalation, the increases being almost twice those measured in age-matched controls. Furthermore, during the headache interval CO_2 responsiveness was lessened or lost. Another interesting observation was that, although in normal volunteers the CBF increase to hypercapnia was symmetrical throughout the brain, in patients with migraine the response was asymmetrical with greater vasomotor instability on the side of the most recent and frequent headaches.

This excessive and asymmetrical cerebral vasodilator response to 5-percent CO_2 inhalation was then used to investigate pharmacological responses of the cerebral circulation in migraine. This might lead to better understanding of the hemicranial nature of the pain of migraine, which has been known since antiquity (the name migraine is derived from the ancient term "hemicrania").

Since Wolff had shown abnormal extracranial vascular responses to catecholamines during the headache and interheadache phases of migraine, we decided to test the hypothesis that there might be an abnormality of the cerebrovascular adrenoceptor sites in both migraine and cluster headache [6].

We systematically studied the rCBF responses in 92 patients with different types of headache [7]: 20 patients with classic migraine, 4 with complicated migraine, 5 with basilar migraine, 37 with common migraine, 11 with cluster headache, and 15 with muscle contraction headache.

Drugs selected for testing were those commonly used in migraine, well-known for their pharmacological properties. All were given by mouth between rCBF measurements. Isometheptene (Midrin) was used as a peripherally acting alpha-receptor stimulator. Dihydroergotoxine (Hydergine) was used as a peripheral alpha-receptor blocker. Isoproterenol (Isuprel) was selected as the beta-receptor stimulator, and propranolol (Inderal) as the beta-receptor blocker. Finally, clonidine (Catapres) was selected as the centrally acting alpha-blocker. Three to four serial measurements of rCBF were made in each patient: the first in the steady state and/or during CO_2 administration prior to any medication, the next in the steady state after oral administration of the drug, and the last during CO_2 inhalation after ingestion of the drug. Results were compared with those in normal volunteers and in patients with muscle contraction headache.

Unlike the responses in patients with vascular headache, no abnormal cerebral vasomotor responses were noted in patients with muscle contraction headaches. In those patients, cerebral vasodilator responses to 5-percent CO_2 inhalation were found to be the same as responses measured in age-matched normal volunteers so they provided excellent controls. Oral administration of the alpha-adrenoceptor stimulator isometheptene to patients during muscle contraction headaches produced no significant change (Figure 3).

Patients with migraine and cluster headache, however, showed significant asymmetrical reductions of rCBF after oral administration of the alpha-stimulator isometheptene, the greatest reduction of rCBF being measured on the side of the most recent headache (Figure 3). Greatest reductions resulted when the medication was administered during the headache interval, and, as rCBF decreased, the vast majority of patients concurrently reported prompt relief of their headache. Patients classified as having basilar migraine, because of symptoms attributable to ischemia in the territory of the basilar artery, showed maximal reductions of rCBF in the brainstem-cerebellar regions.

Oral administration of the alpha-adrenoceptor blocker dihydroergotoxine provided further pharmacological confirmation of the asymmetrical disorders of cerebral alpha-adrenoceptor sites in migraineurs. When the medication was given during the headache-free interval, there were significant but asymmetric increases of hemispheric blood flow which were maximal on the side of the most recent headache.

The receptor-site disorder in migraine was considered as most probably caused by denervation hypersensitivity, as oral administration of the centrally acting alpha-blocker, clonidine, produced less remarkable rCBF increases in the opposite hemisphere than did the peripherally acting blocker, dihydroergotoxine. In other words, when clonidine was given, the hemisphere on the side of the most recent headache showed less vasodilation than the nonheadache hemisphere (Figure 2A, B).

In keeping with a possible sympathetic denervation hypersensitivity disorder, the adrenoceptor site overactivity seems to involve beta- as well as alpha-receptors. Oral administration of isoproterenol produced an asymmetric increase of rCBF greater on the side of the most recent headache. Chronic beta-blockage by oral administration of propranolol to migraineurs reduced the severity and frequency of headaches; during the headache interval rCBF increases were less than expected when compared to age-matched controlled migraineurs who were not taking any medication during the headache phase.

MEASUREMENTS OF rCBF

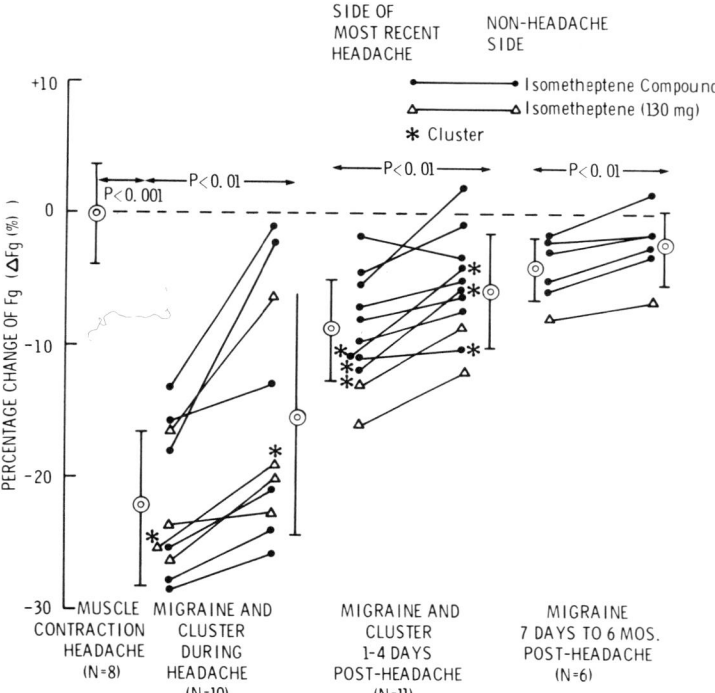

Figure 3. Summary of results of pharmacological testing with α-adrenoceptor stimulator isometheptene (Midrin). rCBF changes in each hemisphere (headache vs. nonheadache side) are compared. As shown at left, there is no change in rCBF in patients with muscle contraction headache. During migraine and cluster headache there is greater reduction on side of most recent headache. As headache subsides, and between headaches, excessive asymmetrical response is less marked but still present. (Modified after Yamamoto M, Meyer S [7].)

Administration of the above-noted peripherally acting alpha- and beta-blockers and stimulators tended to restore excessive CO_2 responsiveness toward normal in patients with migraine, but this was not the case with the centrally acting alpha-receptor blocker, clonidine.

The excessive cerebral vasodilator response to 5-percent CO_2 inhalation in patients with migraine seems most likely to be caused by excessive responses of cerebral vascular adrenoceptor sites, as reduction of the sensitivity of receptor sites to epinephrine and norepinephrine has been shown to occur during hypercapnia [8–11]. This disorder may well be the result of a partial denervation of regional adrenoceptor sites, and it may be related to a genetically determined vasomotor instability among migraineurs.

Acknowledgment

This work was supported by USPHS grant NS09287, Baylor Center for Cerebrovascular Research.

REFERENCES

1. Meyer JS, Ishihara N, Deshmukh VC, Naritomi H, Sakai F, Pollack P: An improved method for non-invasive measurement of regional cerebral blood flow by ^{133}Xe inhalation. *Stroke* 9:195–210, 1978.
2. Obrist W, Thompson HK Jr, Wang HS, Wilkinson WE: Regional cerebral blood flow estimated by ^{133}Xenon inhalation. *Stroke* 6:245–256, 1975.
3. Bickerstaff ER: Basilar artery migraine. *Lancet* 2:15, 1961.
4. Sakai F, Meyer JS: Regional cerebral hemodynamics during migraine and cluster headaches measured by the ^{133}Xe inhalation method. *Headache* 18:122–132, 1978.
5. Wolff HG: *Headache and Other Head Pain*, 2nd Edition. New York, Oxford University Press, 1962.
6. Sakai F, Meyer JS: Abnormal cerebrovascular reactivity in patients with migraine and cluster headache. *Headache* 19:257–266, 1979.
7. Yamamoto M, Meyer JS: Hemicranial disorder of vasomotor adrenoceptors in migraine and cluster headache. *Headache* 20:321–335, 1980.
8. Bygdeman S, Von Euler NS: The effect of respiratory acidosis upon the peripheral vascular reactivity of noradrenaline in the cat. *Acta Physiol Scand* 54:138–146, 1972.
9. Edvinsson L, Aubineau P, Owman C, Sercombe R, Seylaz J: Sympathetic innervation of cerebral arteries. Prejunctional supersensitivity to norepinephrine of sympathectomy or cocaine treatment. *Stroke* 6:525–530, 1975.
10. Wahl M, Kuchinsky W, Bosse O, Oleson J, Lassen NA, Lugvar DH, Michaelis J: Effect of L-norepinephrine on the diameter of pial arterioles and arteries in the cat. *Circ Res* 31:248–256, 1972.
11. *Neurogenic Control of the Brain Circulation*. Wenner-Gren Center International Symposium Series, vol. 30. Owman C and Edvinsson L. (eds). New York, Pergamon Press, 1977.

Chapter 2
Complicated Migraine and Differential Diagnosis of Migraine

NINAN T. MATHEW, M.D.

COMPLICATED MIGRAINE

Complicated migraine is defined as migraine headaches associated with transient, reversible (or, rarely, persistent) visual, ocular, neurological, and psychic symptoms and signs. By definition, there is bound to be an overlap between complicated migraine and classical migraine with its transient visual and neurological prodromes. Complicated migraine is classified in Table 1.

General Characteristics of Complicated Migraine

In the majority of patients, the onset of complicated migraine occurs before age 25 and the attack pattern usually is stereotyped. The frequency of attacks is lower than in the usual migraine syndrome. It is not unusual for a person with previous uncomplicated migraine to develop a complicated migraine, nor is it rare for the complicated migraine to cease and be replaced by migraine without neurological symptoms.

Neurological, visual, and psychic symptoms may precede, accompany, or follow the headache attack. The duration of symptoms may vary from 20 minutes to many days. In rare cases, the occurrence of neurological symptoms may be totally dissociated in time to the headache, making the diagnosis difficult.

Table 1

Complicated Migraine

1. *Ocular complications*
   Persistent field defects
   Ophthalmoplegic migraine
   Ophthalmic migraine
2. *Hemiplegic migraine*
   Hemiplegic and hemisensory disturbances
   Familial hemiplegic migraine
3. *Basilar artery migraine (Bickerstaff)*
4. *Migraine with alterations in higher functions*
   Transient global amnesia
   Migraine stupor
   Confusional state
   Miscellaneous mental reactions, e.g., hallucinations
5. *Dysarrhythmic migraine*

Ocular Complications

Persistent field defects

Persistent scotoma or hemianopic field defects have been reported [1, 2]. Permanent field defects may result from damage to either the retina or the visual cortex in patients exhibiting homonymous hemianopic defects.

Ophthalmoplegic migraine

Ophthalmoplegic migraine is a rare type of migraine that may occur in the young adult. Of 1219 cases of migraine analyzed at the Houston Headache Clinic only one patient was found to have been diagnosed as having ophthalmoplegic migraine. Third-nerve paralysis may occur on the same side as the headache, the paralysis developing after the headache subsides. Duration of the paralysis ranges from hours to days and, if migraine attacks recur, the paralysis may become permanent. Both internal and external ophthalmoplegia may occur. The differential diagnosis of this condition is important; it includes internal carotid or posterior communicating arterial aneurysms, Tolossa-Hunt syndrome, and diabetic ophthalmoplegia. These conditions will be discussed later in this chapter.

Ophthalmic migraine

The term ophthalmic migraine is used generally to denote the condition of patients who present with recurrent visual disturbance without accompanying headaches. In three such patients seen at the Houston Headache Clinic in the past three years, the visual disturbances consisted of hemianopic defect with scintillating scotoma, lasting an average of 20 to 30 minutes. All were women, aged 19, 28 and 34 who had a family history of migraine. Neurological tests including electroencephalograms, computed axial tomography (CAT) scans, and arteriograms were negative. The 19-year-old patient responded to propanolol with a reduced number of attacks, and she was able to stop taking the medication eventually. The 28-year-old woman, who had had her first migraine episode during pregnancy and a series of attacks during the first three months after delivery, developed classical migraine in subsequent months. In the 34-year-old woman, the fourth attack was accompanied by a unilateral throbbing headache even though the first three were unassociated with headache.

When ophthalmic migraine occurs in individuals older than 50 years, it has to be differentiated from amaurosis fugax, which is a manifestation of transient ischemic attacks (Table 2).

Hemiplegic Migraine

Patients with hemiplegic migraine experience unilateral motor or sensory deficit in relation to a migraine attack. Paralysis usually is incom-

Table 2

Ophthalmic Migraine versus Amaurosis Fugax

	Ophthalmic Migraine	Amaurosis Fugax
Duration	10–30 minutes	2–5 minutes
Location	hemianopic	monocular
Visual loss	variable	total or partial
Scotoma	scintillating fortification spectra	photopsias
Bruit	none	carotid bruit may be present
Family history of migraine	++	none
Risk factors for cerebrovascular disease	none	+++

plete and is succeeded by unilateral headaches, nausea, vomiting, and malaise. Weakness may last for hours or days after the headache has subsided. During repeated attacks weakness recurs always on the same side. A familial form of hemiplegic migraine, in which many family members have recurrent headaches and weakness of the same side of the body, has been reported.

Figure 1 shows a CAT brain scan of a 47-year-old patient with an 18-year history of migraine. Three episodes of hemiparetic migraine left her with hemiparetic weakness lasting from 5 to 10 days. The scan, done on the ninth day after the onset of headache, shows a large section of low density in the parietal area. In follow-up scans the low-density area had disappeared. It was presumed to be an area of ischemic cerebral edema, which accounted for the patient's hemiparesis. Fatal infarction of the brain has been reported in migraine [3].

Basilar Artery Migraine

Bickerstaff [4–6] in the early 1960s described a distinctive form of complicated migraine characterized by neurologic signs, including abrupt loss of consciousness, referable to the brainstem. Occurring most often in young women, the syndrome's cardinal manifestations consist of a variety of brainstem, cerebellar, and occipital cortical symptoms, generally in association with usual symptoms of migraine. When there is loss of consciousness, it is invariably brief and akinetic. Protracted confusional epi-

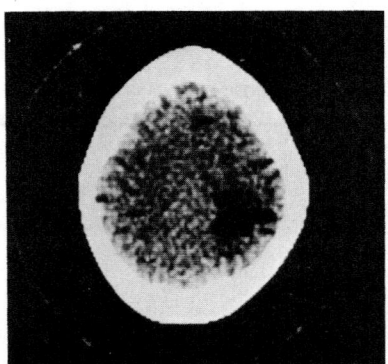

Figure 1. CAT scan of brain showing low-density area in parietal region.

sodes, a common manifestation of juvenile migraine [7], may occur. Table 3 shows the clinical characteristics of nine patients with basilar artery migraine whom I have examined in recent years.

Transient global amnesia [8], migraine stupor [9], confusional states [7], and other distant disturbances in higher functions may be the presenting features of certain patients with complicated migraine. Transient ischemia of vertebrobasilar arterial territory has been considered to be the cause of such manifestations.

DIFFERENTIAL DIAGNOSIS OF MIGRAINE

A number of conditions that cause acute and chronic recurrent headache come under the differential diagnosis of migraine.

Common neurological disorders in which headache is a prominent symptom are given in Table 4 [10].

Table 3

Clinical Summary of Nine Cases of Patients with Basilar Artery Migraine

Clinical Features	Number
Female	9
Male	0
Ages	15–29
Age of onset	before 22 in all
Nausea, vomiting, photophobia	9
Ataxia	9
Vertigo	4
Tinnitus	4
Parasthesia, facial	5
limb	6
Diplopia	4
Confusional episode	2
Loss of consciousness	7—brief—akinetic
Convulsion	0
EEG abnormality	3 (mild dysarrhythmia)

Table 4

Classification of Conditions That Cause Headache

MENINGEAL IRRITATION

Subarachnoid hemorrhage
    Intracranial aneurysm
    Arteriovenous malformation
Meningitis
Meningoencephalitis
Postpneumoencephalographic reaction

TRACTION OR DISPLACEMENT OF INTRACRANIAL PAIN-SENSITIVE STRUCTURES

Space-occupying lesions
  brain tumors, cysts
  brain abscess
  hematomas: extradural, subdural, intracerebral
Increased intracranial pressure
  secondary to space-occupying lesion
  secondary to obstruction of cerebrospinal fluid pathways (hydroencephalus)
  benign intracranial hypertension
Reduced intracranial pressure
  after lumbar puncture
  after ventriculoatrial and ventriculoperitoneal shunt
  posttraumatic and postsurgical tear of meninges and cerebrospinal fluid leakage

SIMPLE INTRACRANIAL VASODILATION

Medications
  nitrites
  histamines
Circulating toxins
  acute infections, febrile illness
  foreign protein reactions
  "hangover" headache
  caffeine withdrawal
Metabolic
  hypoxia: chronic pulmonary insufficiency, high altitude
  hypercapnia: chronic pulmonary insufficiency, Pickwickian syndrome, extreme obesity
  hypoglycemia: insulin-induced, spontaneous
Postconcussional
Postconvulsive
Acute cerebrovascular insufficiency—transient ischemic attacks
Acute hypertensive reactions
  acute nephritis
  pheochromocytoma

tyramine ingestion by a patient taking monoamine oxidase inhibitors
hypertensive encephalopathy
Headache in hypertensive patients
Cough headache and effort or exertional headache of benign etiology

CRANIAL NERVE DISORDERS

Compression of cranial nerves
Trigeminal and glossopharyngeal neuralgia
Extreme stimulation (ice cream headache)

HEADACHE CAUSED BY INFLAMMATION OF CRANIAL STRUCTURES

Arteritis—temporal arteritis
Headache due to inflammation or infection of ocular, aural, nasal and sinus, dental or other cranial or neck structures
Tolossa-Hunt syndrome

A proper history must be obtained, detailed physical and neurological examination made and, whenever indicated, a neurological workup done before the diagnosis of migraine is made. In the remaining portions of this chapter the common clinical conditions that produce headache as a prominent and sometimes as the only symptom will be discussed with an attempt to bring out their differential characteristics from those of migraine.

Subarachnoid Hemorrhage

Intracranial aneurysm and arteriovenous malformation form the majority of causes of subarachnoid hemorrhage.

Intracranial Aneurysms

Unruptured intracranial aneurysms

Unruptured intracranial aneurysms usually are asymptomatic and not associated with headaches. Aneurysms in special locations can, however, be associated with recurring headaches. Those arising from the posterior communication artery, for example, may cause head pain in about 20 percent of patients prior to the subarachnoid hemorrhage. Another special site is the intracavernous aneurysm which usually becomes large and may be associated with progressive unilateral pain in the region of the eye or behind the eye, precipitated by activity. Generally, to rule out conditions like aneurysms or tumors, one should look for such other signs of neurological involvement as ocular paralysis in any patient with strictly unilateral recurrent headaches. Incidence of migraine in patients with intracranial aneurysms is about 5 to 6 percent, not very different from that of the general population.

Ruptured intracranial aneurysms

When an intracranial aneurysm ruptures, there is invariably a sudden and acute onset of headache. The diagnosis of a ruptured aneurysm may be made without much difficulty in the majority of patients. Points that will aid in diagnosing an acute ruptured aneurysm are: (1) Explosive onset of extremely severe headache. (2) Associated signs of meningeal irritation such as neck stiffness and Kernig's sign. (3) Other neurological symptoms and signs such as altered consciousness, oculomotor paralysis, or paresis of the extremities. (4) Uniformly blood-stained cerebral spinal fluid. Spinal tap is a must in diagnosis of subarachnoid hemorrhage. Of course, any spinal fluid containing blood must be differentiated from a traumatic tap. (5) CAT scan will aid in diagnosis. If there is much blood in the subarachnoid space, it can be identified with such a scan. Moderate- and large-sized aneurysms can be identified by the CAT scan, especially after contrast injection. (6) A cerebral arteriogram is diagnostic. It will show the location of the aneurysm, the presence of cerebral vasospasm and, in occasional cases, space-occupying cerebral hematomas.

Clinical features pointing to presence of arteriovenous malformation of the brain

These are: (1) Migraine headaches always on the same side. (2) Visual disturbances always in the opposite half of the visual field. (3) Focal cerebral seizures. (4) Hemiparesis or hemianopsia outlasting the headache. (5) Intracranial bruit. (6) Previous history of intracranial bleeding.

In a typical classical migraine, even though it is usually unilateral, there may be switching of the sides with subsequent attacks, whereas in migraine headache associated with arteriovenous malformation the headache is always in the same location. Even though the physician's chances of hearing an intracranial bruit are slim, routine auscultation of the head may be worthwhile in examining a headache patient. Figure 2 shows a large arteriovenous malformation in a patient who also has recurrent migraine.

Headache Associated with Space-Occupying Lesions: Brain Tumors

The headache associated with brain tumor may be mild, severe, or absent, depending upon the tumor's site of origin. Headache is one of the

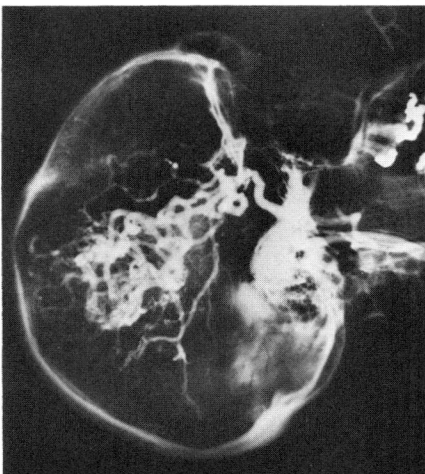

Figure 2. Parietal arteriovenous malformation in a patient who also has recurrent symptoms of classical migraine.

cardinal signs of brain tumor, particularly of rapidly expanding tumors which produce traction on the pain-sensitive structures of the head. This is especially so if the ventricular system is compromised by obstruction of absorption or flow of cerebrospinal fluid, causing hydrocephalus. Headache with increased intracranial pressure is sometimes a prominent finding. But with more slowly growing tumors, headache may be transitory or mild, or easily relieved by common analgesics, and the patient's description of the head pain in this situation may be low-key. The most severe head pain is not usually related to tumor but to vascular headaches or severe neuralgia. Below are some generalizations concerning headache to aid in the localization of brain tumors in patients:

1. Although the headache associated with brain tumor may be referred from a distant intracranial source, the headache approximately overlies the tumor in about one-third of patients.
2. If the tumor is above the tentorium, the pain frequently is at the vertex, or in the frontal regions.
3. If the tumor is below the tentorium, the pain is occipital, and cervical muscle spasm may be present.
4. Headache is almost always present with posterior fossa tumor.

5. If the tumor is midline, it may be increased with coughing, straining, or sudden head movement. (This also occurs with migraine.)
   6. If the tumor is hemispheric, the pain is usually felt on the same side of the head.
   7. If the tumor is chiasmal, at the sella, the pain may be referred to the vertex.

Quality and intensity of brain-tumor headache

Brain-tumor headache is usually intermittent, but in one-tenth of patients it is continuous. The headache is sometimes severe, but rarely is it as intense as that of migraine or the headache associated with ruptured cerebral aneurysm, meningitis, or certain febrile illnesses, or that induced by certain drugs. It is usually relieved by acetylsalicylic acid, or cold packs applied to the scalp, both indications of its moderate intensity. The headache rarely interferes with sleep. It is aggravated by coughing, or straining at stool, and sometimes it is worse in the erect than in the recumbent position. It is also commonly aggravated by the onset of a minor infection. If there is any variation in intensity during the 24-hour cycle, it is worse in the early morning.

Even when the tumor directly compresses or extensively stretches the cranial nerves containing pain afferents, the pain is not as intense as that of tic douloureux, and indeed is often mild or absent.

Unless the pain is severe, nausea with tumor headache is slight. Vomiting may occur with displacement or compression of the medulla and be sometimes "projectile," perhaps because it is unexpected when unaccompanied by nausea. The headache, when occipital or suboccipital, is sometimes associated with stiffness or aching of the muscles of the neck and tilting of the head toward the side of the tumor.

Various types of tumors in relation to headache

Unless a tumor or cyst occupies a strategic position along the line of the cerebrospinal fluid pathway of the ventricles, it may attain considerable size before causing headache. Infiltrating gliomas which remain intracerebral may grow large and occupy a major portion of a cerebral hemisphere without causing headache, because the pain-sensitive structures may remain undisturbed. Rather than producing headache, these tumors are more likely to produce focal or generalized seizures, focal paralysis, progressive or other intellectual impairment, or other neurologic deficit in the initial stages of the disease. A sudden onset of severe headache, with worsening of already existing neurologic deficit or development of neurologic symptoms for the first time, may be seen in patients with some tumors like glioblastoma multiforme, because of bleeding into the tumor area or thrombosis of a major cerebral vein with subsequent cerebral infarction.

Localized swelling and tenderness may be seen at the side of a meningioma. The mastoid area may show slight swelling and tenderness in case of a cerebellopontine angle tumor.

With certain tumors of the third ventricle the headache may come on paroxysmally. In such patients, changes of head position, particularly bending over or lying down, may initiate severe headache. This has been explained by the ball-valve action of the tumor.

In patients with posterior fossa tumors, headache is a prominent early symptom, with pain referred to the occipital region and posterior aspect of the neck. However, intramedullary tumors of the brainstem, especially brainstem gliomae, may progress with other neurologic signs and without headache.

Headache is an early manifestation of tumors of the upper brainstem region, especially pinealomas. The pain is caused by early obstruction of the aqueduct of Sylvius and development of increased intracranial pressure.

Tumors in and around the pituitary gland usually cause bilateral frontoretroorbital and temporal headache which initially may be mild and intermittent. As the tumor expands the headache may become continuous and bursting in character. Usually endocrine changes, visual impairment, optic nerve changes, and changes in the sella turcica seen plainly by x-ray make the diagnosis fairly easy.

Occipital-lobe tumors may give rise to headache associated with vomiting and visual hallucinations in the homonymous visual field, simulating migraine. Careful neurologic examination will reveal a persistent homonymous visual field defect between attacks, and serial examination will show the progressive nature of the problem, unlike migraine.

The symptoms of cerebral abscess are essentially like those of any expanding lesion of the brain. Headache is an early symptom. Fever, nausea, vomiting, and focal convulsion occur frequently. Increased intracranial pressure with papilledema may develop in a few days.

Because of the extensive cerebral edema associated with the development of a cerebral abscess, electroencephalographic abnormalities in the nature of focal slow waves develop early. This is helpful in suspecting a cerebral abscess.

Subdural Hematoma

Headache is one of the common symptoms of both acute and chronic subdural hematoma. The most common cause of subdural hematoma, trauma, however, may seem insignificant or remote to the patient, who may totally ignore it while giving a history. Some spontaneous subdural hematomas do occur. Certain patients vulnerable to subdural hematoma are the elderly, chronic alcoholics, patients taking anticoagulants, patients with blood dyscrasias, and patients with systemic malignancy. Although headache usually is a symptom of the condition, other prominent symptoms and signs may mask the headache totally, and those need to be recognized. Altered consciousness and drowsiness, confusion and disorientation, and progressive dementia may be the most prominent symptoms in chronic subdural hematoma, especially in elderly persons. Signs of brain herniation may be evident in advanced cases. Papilledema may be present in the chronic variety.

Intracerebral Hematoma

Other intracranial hemorrhagic problems, mostly acute in nature, may be associated with headache. Common sites of intracerebral hemorrhage are the external capsule and thalamus, pons, and cerebellum. The headaches associated with acute intracerebral hematoma and intracerebral hemorrhage are severe and sudden in onset, usually associated with rapidly progressing alteration in consciousness or development of dense neurological deficit such as hemiparesis. The neurological symptoms and signs vary with the location of the hematoma. A pontine hemorrhage produces sudden and total loss of consciousness with pupillary abnormalities and signs of quadriparesis. Cerebellar hemorrhage causes sudden, severe occipital headache associated with abnormal eye movements, irregular breathing, and paralysis of the extremities. A CAT scan of the brain is highly diagnostic of most intracranial hemorrhages; the technique has brought considerable improvement to diagnostic accuracy of intracerebral hematomas. A great majority of these patients are severely hypertensive.

Increased Intracranial Pressure

Headache is the most common symptom of an increase in intracranial pressure, which may be caused by space-occupying intracranial lesions such as tumors, cysts, or hematomas; obstruction of cerebrospinal fluid pathways producing hydrocephalus; or benign intracranial hypertension.

Obstruction of cerebrospinal fluid pathways

Any lesion that obstructs the flow of cerebrospinal fluid from the lateral ventricle through the foramen of Monro, third ventricle, sylvian aqueduct, fourth ventricle, and its exit foramina, or prevents the passage of cerebrospinal fluid over the cortex to its absorption sites will cause a rapid increase in intracranial pressure so that headache becomes the main presenting symptom. Cysts of the third ventricle, especially colloid cysts, tumors encroaching on the posterior part of the third ventricle such as pinealomas, congenital stenosis of the aqueduct, and obstruction of the aqueduct and fourth ventricle by tumors arising from the fourth ventricle, such as an ependymoma, are usual causes of hydrocephalus. Adhesive arachnoiditis caused by chronic meningitis, which blocks the exit foramina and the subarachnoid space near the sylvian areas, and such congenital malformations in the posterior fossa as Dandy-Walker syndrome and Arnold-Chiari malformation produce obstruction to cerebrospinal fluid pathways.

Stenosis of the aqueduct usually is a congenital malformation which is asymptomatic until some systemic infection causes proliferation of the ependymal lining, which then blocks the canal and produces an acute internal hydrocephalus. Communicating hydrocephalus may form after subarachnoid hemorrhage, head injury, and some forms of meningitis caused by obstruction of cerebrospinal fluid pathways near the cerebral convexities.

Headache is the most common presenting symptom, with pain more or less constant and usually worse on awakening. The headache is diffuse and aggravated by coughing or sneezing. As the intracranial pressure increases, nausea, vomiting, and visual disturbances may develop. Diplopia caused by paralysis of unilateral or bilateral lateral rectus muscle is seen in severe cases. Sixth-nerve paralysis usually is a false localizing sign in these patients. Papilledema develops fairly early in obstructive hydrocephalus and, if untreated, will go on to secondary optic atrophy and result in permanent visual impairment. Ataxia of gait is a common sign of rapidly developing hydrocephalus. Restriction of upward gaze may also be seen in some patients as a nonspecific sign, even though it is considered pathognomonic of a pinealoma. Figure 3 shows a CAT scan demonstrating the presence of obstructive hydrocephalus of fairly rapid onset as a result of adhesive arachnoiditis in a young patient who presented with increasingly severe headaches and ataxia over a period of a few weeks. The clinical manifestation of a congenital aqueductal stenosis may occur for the first time in adult life when a patient presents with a progressive headache.

X-rays of the skull are helpful because of the changes in the sella as a result of increased intracranial pressure. The sella enlarges with demineralization of its processes and walls, and eventual destruction. Changes also are observed in the cranial vault. Separation of the sutures is invariably seen in children with internal hydrocephalus. One may have to resort

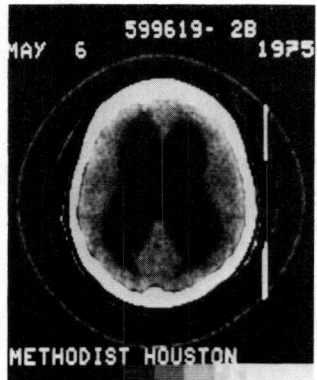

Figure 3. CAT scan of brain showing enormous enlargement of lateral ventricles in patient with acute obstructive hydrocephalus.

to a pneumoencephalogram in some cases to arrive at an etiologic diagnosis of the hydrocephalus. This is especially true in some patients with third-ventricular obstruction, aqueductal stenosis, obstruction to the exit foramina of the fourth ventricle, and obstruction of the passage of cerebrospinal fluid to the convex areas of the brain.

Benign intracranial hypertension

Pseudotumor cerebri and otitic hydrocephalus are synonyms for this condition.

The condition is referred to as benign intracranial hypertension because of its relatively benign course and the relative well-being of the patient. The majority of patients are young or middle-aged, moderately obese women who have some menstrual irregularities. Apart from constant, unremitting headache, the patient does not usually have other complaints. Neurologic examination invariably reveals papilledema without any focal neurologic abnormalities. The patient generally looks healthy and well. If left untreated, the papilledema may lead to secondary optic atrophy and consequent visual loss. Occasionally sixth-nerve paresis may develop. Even though in the majority of patients this is a self-limiting disease, a chronic form is not uncommon.

A patient who presents with headache and papilledema should be examined thoroughly to exclude other intracranial processes. In benign intracranial hypertension, skull x-rays and the electroencephalogram are normal. Next step is a CAT scan of the brain, which usually reveals a relatively small ventricular system without other abnormality. No enlargement of ventricles or displacement is found, unlike with other causes of intracranial hypertension. Pneumoencephalography and arteriography reveal a "pinched" appearance of the lateral ventricles without other abnormality. Obstruction of the lateral or sigmoid venous sinuses may be detected in the last phases of cerebral arteriogram. Once a space-occupying lesion is excluded from the diagnosis, a spinal tap may be done safely; this will reveal very high intracranial pressure, usually from 300 to 500 mm H_2O. Cerebrospinal fluid cell count and chemistry are normal, and cerebrospinal fluid is sterile.

Treatment for the condition mainly aims at reducing the intracranial pressure. Furosemide (Lasix), acetazolamide (Diamox), and other diuretics have been used, as have corticosteroids and long-term prescription of oral glycerol. If medical treatment fails and if a secondary optic atrophy threatens to develop, subtemporal decompression may be indicated. Some neurosurgeons prefer a lumbartheco-peritoneal shunt.

Reduced intracranial pressure following lumbar puncture, ventriculoatrial and ventriculoperitoneal shunt, and cerebrospinal fluid leakage from trauma or surgical treatment of meninges may cause headache. Puncture of the subarachnoid space for the introduction of air, anesthetic, radiographic contact material, radioactive materials, or steroids may produce headache. Leakage of the cerebrospinal fluid through the dural-arachnoidal puncture hole brings about a dilation of intracranial vessels and traction on the blood vessels.

Headache occurs within hours after lumbar puncture in about 32 percent of patients, the pain varying with postural changes. The headache is most severe when the patient is upright and is relieved when he or she lies down. The headache is bifrontal or bioccipital, but it may involve the entire head. Headache usually begins 6 to 48 hours after the spinal puncture and may last for a number of days; in some patients it lasts for 2 to 3 weeks. The size of the needle used, amount of fluid withdrawn, and multiple punctures are factors that influence the development of postlumbar puncture headache.

Headache in Ischemic Cerebrovascular Disease

About 25 percent of transient ischemic attacks (TIA) are associated with headache. Headaches often accompany the ischemic event, but they sometimes precede it by days, weeks, or months and then may or may not accompany the eventual stroke or TIA. In patients with multiple strokes or TIAs, headaches may occur with some episodes and not with others.

Individual headaches may last minutes or hours, sometimes days. The duration of headache bears no relation to the severity of vascular disease, degree of ischemia, or its outcome. The quality of headache varies; some patients describe it as throbbing, others as steady. The intensity varies also, ranging from barely noticeable to discomfort so severe that cerebral hemorrhage may be suspected. The majority of headaches are, however, mild to moderate.

The headaches associated with ischemic cerebrovascular disease usually are ipsilateral to the diseased vessel, anterior when the disease involves the internal carotid artery or its branches, and posterior when the vertebrobasilar system is involved. Exceptions are common. A frequent variation, for example, is the occurrence of bifrontal headaches in vertebrobasilar disease.

When transient ischemic attacks that produce neurological signs and symptoms are associated with headache, it may be important to differentiate the headache from complicated migraine, which also could produce transient neurological symptomatology. A number of differentiating features will enable the physician to determine whether a given case is a transient ischemic attack with headache or a complicated migraine. In transient ischemic attacks with headaches, the headaches are brief and they usually precede the neurological symptoms. Previous history of migraines as well as family history of migraine will be helpful in differentiating the two conditions. Identifying risk factors for cerebrovascular disease and carotid or vertebral bruit might be of additional benefit in differentiating TIAs with headache from complicated migraine.

Temporal Arteritis

Temporal arteritis affects more women than men, in the ratio of 7:4, most patients being over age 50 although one 35-year-old patient has been reported. Such symptoms of systemic disturbance as weight loss, night sweats, aching of joints, and low-grade fever are commonly associated, merging into the syndrome known as "polymyalgia rheumatica."

Most patients complain of head pains or headache, unilateral or bilateral, which may be localized to the affected scalp vessels. Pain in the jaw muscles upon chewing is a pathognomonic symptom; it is caused by intermittent claudication of the masseter as a result of narrowing of the extracranial arteries. The disorder also may involve intracranial vessels, particularly the ophthalmic artery, causing blindness from retinal ischemia and subsequent optic atrophy. The aorta, coronary, renal, and iliac arteries have been implicated in some cases.

Typical temporal arteritis starts with pain over the affected scalp arteries which thicken and cease to pulsate. They are usually tender when touched and the skin overlying them may redden. About 20 percent of untreated patients lose their vision in one or both eyes.

Apart from obvious changes in the scalp vessels, the physical signs vary according to the extent of involvement of the cerebral and other arteries. The ophthalmoscopic picture of central retinal artery thrombosis may be seen, retinal ischemia and edema with dimpling in the macular region producing a grayish-red spot. At a later stage the optic disc becomes atrophic.

The erythrocyte sedimentation rate (ESR) is higher than 45 mm/h in most patients and ranges up to 120 mm/h. Electrophoresis of serum proteins demonstrates increase in alpha- and beta-globulin fractions. Most patients have a mild hypochromic anemia and polymorphonuclear leucocytosis. Biopsy of the temporal artery (or the facial artery if this is more appropriate to the site of pain) shows thickening of the intima, fibrosis and cellular infiltration of the vessel wall, often with giant cells resembling those of tuberculous disease or arcoidosis, and thrombus formation in the lumen.

Early diagnosis is of great importance. When the condition is suspected based on the patient's clinical history, whether or not the ESR is elevated, a temporal artery should be biopsied. Treatment with steroids may be started immediately, before the biopsy is taken. Steroid therapy may have to be continued for years, and it is reassuring to have a firm histological diagnosis at the outset.

Tolossa-Hunt Syndrome

This condition produces recurrent ophthalmoplegia accompanied by unilateral pain behind the eye. Paralysis of the third, fourth, sixth, and first division of the fifth cranial nerve usually occurs in varying combinations. Granulomatous inflammation of the superior orbital fissure or cavernous sinus is the usual cause. This condition comes under the differential diagnosis of ophthalmoplegic migraine.

REFERENCES

1. Galezwoski X: Ophthalmic megum. *Lancet* 1:176–177, 1882.
2. Hunt JF: A contribution to the paralytic and other persistent sequelae of migraine. *Am J Med Sci* 150:313–314, 1915.

3. Guest IA, Woolf AL: Fatal infarction of brain in migraine. *Br Med J* 1:225–226, 1964.
4. Bickerstaff ER: Basilar artery migraine. *Lancet* 1:15–17, 1961.
5. Bickerstaff ER: Impairment of consciousness in migraine. *Lancet* 2:1057–1059, 1961.
6. Bickerstaff ER: The basilar artery and the migraine-epilepsy syndrome. *Proc R Soc Med* 55:167–169, 1962.
7. Gascon G, Barlow C: Juvenile migraine presenting as an acute confusional state. *Pediatrics* 45:628–635, 1970.
8. Olivarius BF, Jensen TS: Transient global amnesia in migraine. *Headache* 19:335–338, 1979.
9. Lee CH, Lance JW: Migraine stupor. *Headache* 17:32–38, 1977.
10. Mathew NT: Headache of neurologic origin, in Ryan RE and Ryan RE, Jr (eds): *Headache and Headache Pain and Diagnosis and Treatment*. St. Louis, Mosby, 1978.

Chapter 3
Pharmacological Treatment of Migraine

SEYMOUR DIAMOND, M.D.
JOSE L. MEDINA, M.D.

Treating migraine is not a simple matter. The physician finds himself doing tailoring work week after week. He adds and subtracts medications, not in a haphazard way, but by using his knowledge of the pathogenesis of migraine. We shall review the medications used in the treatment of migraine. The clinician should always remember, however, that a single approach may not be successful and that a combination of drugs directed at different physiopathological mechanisms may be needed. Patients who have migraine need frequent follow-up visits; single consultation is bound to fail.

The pharmacological treatment of migraine may be divided into two categories, preventive and symptomatic.

PREVENTIVE TREATMENT

In preventive treatment the following types of medications are used: antihypertensive drugs, antiserotonergic compounds, antidepressants, and platelet inhibitors.

Antihypertensive Drugs

The most important new contribution to the therapy of migraine was the serendipitous discovery by Rabkin et al. [1] of the disappearance of migraine headaches in a cardiac patient treated with propranolol (Inderal). This incidental medical observation was followed by several published studies. Six of those [2–7] were based on well-controlled double-blind, single cross-over studies in which patients were given daily doses of 80 to 160 mg of propranolol over periods ranging from six weeks to three months.

In one trial a dosage of only 60 mg per day was given to migrainous children weighing less than 35 kg. Propranolol prevented migraine in 55 to 93 percent [2–8] of the patients. These studies, however, were done for short periods of time only. We recently concluded a 14-month study of propranolol, finding the drug to be effective and safe for migrainous patients.

There are several reasons for the effectiveness of propranolol in migraine treatment: (1) propranolol blocks beta receptors and therefore prevents arterial dilatation; (2) it blocks catecholamine-induced platelet aggregation; (3) it decreases platelet adhesiveness; (4) it prevents elevation of coagulation factors during epinephrine release; (5) it shifts the hemoglobin oxygen dissociation curve, promoting release of oxygen to the tissues; (6) it inhibits renine secretion; and (7) it blocks catecholamine-induced lipolysis [9]. The lipolysis inhibition produces a decrease in arachidonic acid, which is a prostaglandin (PG) precursor. The decrease in prostaglandins accounts for the inhibition of platelet aggregation and the diminution of prostaglandins during stress.

If the patient is carefully selected, propranolol is the drug of choice in the prophylaxis of migraine. The patient should not have a history of asthma, chronic obstructive lung disease, congestive heart failure, atrial ventricular conduction disturbances, and should not be under treatment with insulin, hypoglycemic drugs, or monoamine oxidase inhibitors. Propranolol is especially helpful for migraineurs who have severe hypertension, angina pectoris, or thyrotoxicosis for which ergot preparations are contraindicated. In patients free from these conditions, the medication will relieve the headache and coexistent disorders. Another advantage of propranolol over ergot medications is the fact that it does not cause rebound headaches after it is discontinued. Propranolol is taken orally in the dosage of 20 to 40 mg four times a day. In most patients we usually start with 20 mg four times a day for a week and then increase the dosage to 20 mg three times a day, 40 mg at night. The plasma half-life of propranolol is only 2.5 hours. Its beta-blocking action, however, seems to last about 12 hours. Therefore, it may also be effective when it is given twice a day. Propranolol should not be discontinued suddenly by patients with coronary heart disease because withdrawal might exacerbate coronary ischemia and lead to unstable angina or myocardial infarction [10].

Finally, we should be aware of drug interactions. Patients taking hypoglycemic drugs or insulin should not receive propranolol because they might develop hypoglycemia. Hypoglycemia liberates epinephrine, which in turn causes tachycardia and palpitations. All these compensatory and warning mechanisms are blocked by propranolol. Furthermore, as beta receptors in the blood vessels are blocked, alpha receptors predominate and the release of epinephrine may cause severe hypertension.

Another antihypertensive drug used to prevent migraine is clonidine, but there is no consensus concerning its effectiveness. Wilkinson et al. [11] consider clonidine the drug of choice for that 30 percent of migrainous patients who are especially sensitive to tyramine-containing foods. In a short-term study, Stensrud and Sjaastad [12] found clonidine to be effective in 62 percent of patients with migraine headaches, but their long-term study found it effective in only about 40 percent of patients. Shaw and Saunders [13] conducted an eight-month double-blind crossover study with clonidine and placebo and could not demonstrate any significant effects for the drug. Neither could Ryan et al. [14]. We have found clonidine useful in some patients with migraine headaches, but it is not nearly as effective as propranolol. Clonidine acts centrally by inhibiting sympathetic outflow from the vasomotor center in the medulla [15–16], and peripherally by reducing the response of the blood vessels to both constricting and dilating substances [17].

Initial oral dosage of clonidine is 0.1 mg twice a day, which is slowly increased to a maximum of 2.4 mg a day. Abrupt discontinuation of the drug may produce a severe hypertensive crisis and death. The hypertensive crisis is caused by marked increase in the secretion of catecholamines from the adrenal medulla. Therefore, if clonidine has to be discontinued, the dosage should be reduced over a period of two to four days. Side effects with clonidine occur frequently but they are mild. Patients may complain of drowsiness, dryness of mouth, constipation, and an occasional disturbance of ejaculation. Mild orthostatic hypotension occurs in 50 percent of the patients. Depression may be a complication of clonidine treatment. As a matter of fact, tricyclic antidepressants act as inhibitors of clonidine and should not be used in combination. Periodic retinal examinations should be done for patients taking clonidine because retinal degeneration has been reported.

Antiserotonergic Drugs

Cyproheptadine [18] is an antihistamine that works especially well in children with migraine. Its action is caused by its ability to block histamine and serotonin receptors. It is usually given at the dosage of

4 to 12 mg per day. The drug was found to be of value for only 46 percent of adult migraineurs. Besides its low effectiveness in adult patients, the drug has some other actions that make its use for this age group a poor choice. Cyproheptadine often causes drowsiness; it impairs mental performance which results in hazardous driving, and it very frequently causes an increase in appetite and marked weight gain. Children, however, seem to tolerate the medication better, and for them we consider it the medication of choice.

Ergotamine tartrate usually is used in the symptomatic treatment of migraine and it may be indicated in migraine prophylaxis. We find it to be especially useful for menopausal women who are taking high amounts of estrogen because of hot flashes. In these patients Bellergal, a combination of ergotamine tartrate, 0.3 mg, belladonna, 0.1 mg, and phenobarbital, 20 mg, is effective in relieving hot flashes and preventing migraine headaches. This enables the patient to discontinue or markedly reduce the amount of estrogen, thus removing one of the major precipitating factors of migraine. One should be very cautious, however, in using ergotamine daily in high amounts because it may markedly increase the frequency and severity of migraine.

Methysergide [20] may be used as a last resort to treat a patient for severe, intractable migraine headaches. The drug's action is the result of serotonin-blocking; methysergide blocks the vasoconstrictive and inflammatory effects of serotonin. The drug is excreted in the urine and has an eliminating half-life of 2.7 hours although some metabolites are excreted for about 10 hours [21]. Usually it does very little vasoconstricting except in about 2 percent of persons who may develop ischemic complications. In patients who have taken it for a long time, methysergide may cause such fibrotic syndromes as retroperitoneal or endocardial fibrosis [22]. To avoid this, intravenous pyelograms should be done every six months. The drug should be discontinued every six months for at least one month. In addition to these serious side effects, other mild symptoms limit the use of this medication in about one-third of patients. Among these toxic effects are nausea, vomiting, gastrointestinal pain, diarrhea, drowsiness, dizziness, anxiety, hallucinations, and, rarely, psychotic reactions. Muscle cramps, weight gain, and hair loss also are frequently noted.

Methysergide helps about 60 percent of migraine patients; the usual dosage is about 4 to 8 mg per day. It should not be given to pregnant patients or to those with peripheral vascular or coronary artery disease, hypertension, thrombophlebitis, or peptic ulcer.

Pitozifen (Sandomigran) is a drug that has an anti-aminergic effect on serotonin and histamine as well as acetylcholine, tryptamine, and catecholamines. It is usually given at the dosage of 0.5 mg three times a day. After an oral dose of 1 mg, the maximum serum concentration is reached in five to seven hours with minimal activity after 12 hours. The drug is excreted mainly by the kidneys and has a biological half-life of 26 hours. Several European short-term and long-term clinical studies have determined the efficacy of pitozifen in 40 to 68 percent of migraine patients [23-26]. The main side effects of this pill are weight gain, drowsiness, and dizziness. The Food and Drug Administration has not approved the drug in the United States.

A new ergot medication, bromocryptine, is undergoing studies to elevate its efficacy in migraine treatment. Bromocryptine is a semisynthetic ergot alkaloid free of the cardiovascular and oxytoxic actions. Bromocryptine suppresses prolactin [27] and has been successfully used in treatment for premenstrual syndrome [28]. Horrobin [29] observed that migraine is likely to occur at times when prolactin secretion is elevated during periods of stress, oversleeping, premenstruation, and during therapy with estrogen or oral contraceptives. A study of bromocryptine in migrainous patients was done by Hockaday et al. [30] who found a significant improvement of menstrual migraine. They studied 12 menstrual cycles in seven patients; in ten cycles the patients were completely freed of menstrual migraine. The Hockaday group prescribed bromocryptine at the initial dose of 2.5 mg with the evening meal. The dosage was increased to 2.5-mg doses twice a day and then 2.5 mg three times a day at four-day intervals. Among the side effects were nausea, dizziness and light-headedness, leg cramps, gastric discomfort, diarrhea, flatulence, and constipation. We do not believe that a headache that occurs only during the premenstrual or menstrual periods should be treated with a daily drug. Therefore, we have on several occasions prescribed bromocryptine only during the premenstrual and menstrual period but without success.

Antidepressants

In 1970 Anthony and Lance [31] reported on the effect of phenelzine, 45 mg a day, in 25 patients with migraine, 14 of whom had not responded to methysergide, cyproheptadine or ergotamine. At the end of the study 14 patients were considered headache-free or 75 percent improved, six were 50 percent improved, five were unaffected, and six had abandoned treatment. The researchers concluded that monoamine oxidase (MAO) inhibitors are worth trying in patients resistant to other therapies but should be used with extreme caution. We prescribe 45 mg a day of phenelzine for patients who have not responded to any preventive medications.

In the late 1960s amitriptyline was mentioned occasionally for the prophylaxis of migraine, but the medication was not widely used for this purpose until Couch et al. [32] reported its beneficial effect in 1976. These authors, treating 110 patients for severe migraine, found that amitriptyline improved the condition in 72 percent of patients by more than 50 percent, and in 57 percent of patients by more than 80 percent. As the patients' improvement was not related to the drug's antidepressive action, Couch et al. suggested that amitriptyline's other mechanisms of action might be responsible for migraine control. Amitriptyline can block the reuptake of catecholamines and serotonin at nerve endings in both the central and peripheral nervous systems; it has anticholinergic, antihistaminic, and antiserotonergic effects; it may also interfere with the release of norepinephrine at nerve endings. Following the Couch study, a multiclinic double-blind study was undertaken by most of the headache clinics in this country, involving 391 patients with classical or common migraine. The researchers sought to determine whether amitriptyline, 25 to 100 mg per day for 16 weeks, would result in a greater decrease in frequency and severity of migraine headaches than would treatment with placebo. Two hundred patients completed the study. Although the results showed that amitriptyline is not superior to placebo in controlling migraine headaches, we believe that amitriptyline is helpful for patients with mixed migraine and muscle-contraction headaches because many of these patients are depressed.

Platelet Inhibitors

During the past few years the strong relationship found between platelet changes and migraine has evolved into the use of platelet antagonists to prevent the headaches. Among the important platelet changes known to occur in migraine are increased aggregability to serotonin because of the platelet membrane's greater uptake capacity for serotonin [33], chronic hyperaggregability in response to other substances [34–35], and decrease of MAO type B [36].

The migraine attack is initiated by the release of serotonin from platelet [37–38], which may account for the sterile inflammation that occurs in migraine headaches. In addition, elevated platelet adhesiveness during the headache phase parallels the increase in platelet serotonin during the aura phase.

The three major platelet antagonists are aspirin, sulfinpyrazone, and dipyridamol. Aspirin works by inhibiting cyclo-oxygenase, which transforms arachidonic acid to prostaglandin E_2 which subsequently changes to thromboxane. Thromboxane causes platelet aggregation. Aspirin also affects the thrombosthenin of platelets by destroying it [39]. Like aspirin, sulfinpyrazone inactivates cyclo-oxygenase. Dipyridamol works in a different way, inhibiting phosphodiesterase and in this way increasing cyclic adenosine monophosphate (AMP). Cyclic AMP reduces adenosine diphosphate (ADP) release, which is the activity that initiates the chain of events leading to platelet aggregation. Therapeutic dosages of these drugs are 640 to 960 mg of aspirin per day, 400 to 800 mg of sulfinpyrazone per day, and 100 to 400 mg of dipyridamol per day in divided doses. A recent study of aspirin has shown it to be of some benefit in migraine prevention [40]; nine of 12 migraineurs improved with aspirin therapy. The preventive capability of dipyridamol has been studied extensively by Barcia-Marino [41], who found that, of 99 patients, 44 percent responded well to the drug, 23 percent had a moderate response, and the rest showed no effect. Further studies of these drugs are needed to assess their value in migraine prevention.

ABORTIVE TREATMENT

When migraine is mild, the use of aspirin or acetaminophen may be enough to abort the attack. Migraine headaches are usually of moderate to severe intensity, however, and patients rarely respond to such mild medications. The drug of choice in treating migraine attacks is ergotamine tartrate, a vasoconstrictor that is metabolized mainly in the liver. Its elimination half-life is about 6.5 hours, but some metabolites are excreted for 35 hours [21]. The drug's many side effects include abdominal cramps, epigastric discomfort, diarrhea, nausea, vomiting, painful uterine contractions, and seldom intermittent claudication or acute arterial occlusion. Mild side effects such as nausea and vomiting are experienced by about 30 percent of patients, and the more severe toxic effects by about one of 600 patients. Ergotamine may be given orally, sublingually, by inhalation, rectally or parenterally. Oral and sublingual dosages are 2 mg at the onset of the attack and 1 mg every half hour. No more than 6 mg per day or 12 mg per week are allowed. By inhalation, one dose may be taken every four minutes, up to a maximum of six doses per day. Rectally, a 2-mg suppository may be used and repeated one hour later as needed with a maximum of 4 mg per day and 10 mg per week. The recommended dosage for intramuscular or subcutaneous administration is 0.5 to 1.5 mg; maximum dosage allowed is 10 mg per week. The effectiveness of ergotamine is related to the speed with which it is administered [42–44] and the route used. The oral preparation is effective in about one-half of migraine attacks, the sublingual form in 66 percent. Inhalation is effective in about 70 percent, rectal suppositories in 75 percent, and intramuscular injection in about 85 percent. Ergotamine should be administered as soon as the patient feels the headache coming on.

The use of ergotamine is contraindicated in pregnant women, patients with coronary heart disease, peripheral vascular disease, significant hepatic or renal dysfunction, thyrotoxicosis, severe hypertension, sepsis, anemia, Raynaud's phenomenon, and thrombophlebitis.

Dihydroergotamine is a medication whose actions, metabolism, side effects, and indications are similar to ergotamine tartrate. Dihydroergotamine can only be given by the intramuscular route; the usual dosage is 1 mg at the onset of the migraine attack, then hourly up to a maximum daily dosage of 3 mg.

Frequent administration of ergotamine increases the occurrence of migraine because it causes rebound headaches. To avoid these, ergotamine should never be given two days in a row. It is advisable, therefore, not to administer ergotamine to patients who have more than two migraine headaches per week.

Isometheptene mucate is effective in aborting migraine [45]. It is especially useful in patients who cannot tolerate ergotamine or who have peripheral vascular or cardiac disease which would preclude the use of ergotamine. The use of isometheptene is contraindicated in patients who have cardiac and peripheral vascular disease, but its use is much less risky than that of the ergotamines. We consistently use isometheptene in patients who tend to take ergotamine daily and thereby bring on rebound headaches. The drug causes no rebound phenomenon.

Occasionally we treat patients who have prolonged migraine attacks which may last from two to seven days. It is possible that a sterile inflammation has occurred around the vessels participating in the migraine headache. These patients benefit from the use of steroids. Dexamethasone, 16 mg intramuscularly, may be given if the headache does not disappear in the first 24 hours. The drug usually brings dramatic improvement.

REFERENCES

1. Rabkin R, Stables DP, Levin NW: The prophylactic value of propranolol in angina pectoris. *Am J Cardiol* 18:370–383, 1966.
2. Wykes P: The treatment of angina pectoris with coexistent migraine. *Practitioner* 200:702–704, 1968.
3. Bekes M, Matos L, Rausch J, Torok E: Treatment of migraine with propranolol. *Lancet* 2:980, 1968.
4. Weber RG, Reinmuth OM: The treatment of migraine with propranolol. *Neurology* (*Minneap*) 22:366–369, 1972.

5. Malvea BP, Gwon N, Graham JR: Propranolol prophylaxis of migraine. *Headache* 12:163–167, 1973.
6. Diamond S, Medina JL: Double blind study of propranolol for migraine prophylaxis. *Headache* 16:24–27, 1976.
7. Widere T, Vigander T: Propranolol in the treatment of migraine. *Brit M J* 2:699–701, 1974.
8. Ludvigsson J: Propranolol in treatment of migraine in children. *Lancet* 2:799, 1973.
9. Schweizer W: *Beta-Blockers—Present Status and Future Prospects.* Baltimore, University Park Press, 1974.
10. Alderman EL, Coltart J, Wettach GE, Harrison DC: Coronary artery syndromes after sudden propranolol withdrawal. *Ann Intern Med* 81:625–627, 1974.
11. Wilkinson M, Neyian C, Rowsell AR: Clonidine in the treatment of migraine at the city migraine clinic in patients selected with tyramine, in Dalessio DJ, Dalsgaard-Nielsen T, Diamond S: *Proceedings International Headache Symposium.* Basle, Sandoz, 1971, pp 219–221.
12. Stenstrud P, Sjaastad O: Clonidine (Catapresan)—double-blind study after long-term treatment with the drug in migraine. *Acta Neurol Scandinav* 53:233–236, 1976.
13. Shaw DA, Saunders M: A double-blind comparison of Dixarit and placebo. The migraine headache and Dixarit. Proceedings of symposium Churchill College, Cambridge. Bracknell, Berkshire, Boehringer Ingelheim, 1972, pp 54–61.
14. Diamond S, Ryan RE: Double-blind study of clonidine and placebo in the prophylactic treatment of migraine. *Headache* 15:202–206, 1976.
15. Kosman ME: Evaluation of clonidine hydrochloride (Catapres). A new antihypertensive agent. *JAMA* 233:174–175, 1975.
16. Clonidine (Catapres) for hypertension. *The Medical Letter,* May 23, 1975.
17. Fanchamps A: Pharmacodynamic principles of antimigraine therapy. *Headache* 15:79–90, 1975.
18. Douglas WW: Histamine and antihistamines; 5-hydroxytryptamine and antagonists, in Goodman LS, Gilman A (eds): *The Pharmacological Basis of Therapeutics,* 5th Ed. New York, Macmillan, 1975, pp 590–629.
19. Curran DA, Lance SW: Clinical trial of methysergide and other preparations in the management of migraine. *J Neurol Neurosurg Psychiatry* 27:463–469, 1964.
20. Curran DA, Hinterberger H, Lance JW: Methysergide. *Res Clin Stud Headache* 1:74–122, 1967.
21. Meier J, Schreider E: Human plasma levels of some antimigraine drugs. *Headache* 16:96–104, 1976.
22. Graham JR, Suby HI, LeCompte PM, Sudowsky NL: Inflammatory fibrosis associated with methysergide therapy. *Res Clin Stud Headache* 1:123–164, 1967.
23. Pasquazzi M, Anselmi E: C 105 (Sandomigram) nella terapia della emicrania. Esperienza clinica su 30 casi. *Ref MED* 88:267–274, 1974.
24. Sicuteri F, Del Bianco PL, Anselmi B: Migraine as a cyclical disease with latent and overt components—effects of an antaminic drug. *Headache* 10:53–62, 1970.

25. Schaen J: BC-105, a new serotonin antagonist in the treatment of migraine. *Headache* 10:67–73, 1970.
26. Arthur GP, Hornabrook RW: The treatment of migraine with BC-105 (pitozifen): a double-blind trial. *N Z Med J* 464:5–9, 1971.
27. Vaisrub S: The many faces of bromocriptine. *JAMA* 235:2854–2855, 1976.
28. Benedek-Jaszmann LJ, Lequin RM, Sternthal V: Bromocriptine and the premenstrual syndrome. *European Journal of Obstetrics, Gynecology and Reproductive Biology* 5:191–192, 1975.
29. Horrobin DF: *Prolactin: Physiology and Clinical Significance.* Lancaster, Medical and Technical Pub Co Ltd, 1973.
30. Hockaday JM, Peet KMS, Hockaday TDR: Bromocriptine in migraine. *Headache* 16:109–114, 1976.
31. Anthony M, Lance JW: Monoamine oxidase inhibitors in the control of migraine. *Proc Aust Assoc Neurol* 7:45–47, 1970.
32. Couch JR, Ziegler DK, Hassanein R: Amitriptyline in the prophylaxis of migraine. *Neurology (Minneap)* 26:121–127, 1976.
33. Hilton BP: Blood platelets: a pathological difference between migraines and control subjects. *Hemicrania* 3:3–5, 1971.
34. Sandler M: Monoamines and migraine: A path through the woods, in Diamond S, Dalessio DJ, Graham JR, Medina JL (eds): *Vasoactive Substances Relevant to Migraine.* Springfield, Ill, Thomas, 1975, pp 3–18.
35. Lance JW, Anthony M, Gonski A: Serotonin, the carotid body and cranial vessels in migraine. *Arch Neurol* 16:553–558, 1967.
36. Anthony M, Hinterberger H, Lance JW: The possible relationship of serotonin to the migraine syndrome. *Res Clin Stud Headache* 2:29–59, 1969.
37. Deshmukh SV, Meyer JS: Platelet dysfunction in migraine and effect of self-medication with aspirin. *Thromb Haemost* 36:319–324, 1976.
38. Couch JR, Hassanein RS: Platelet aggregability in migraine. *Neurology (Minneap)* 27:643–648, 1977.
39. Caen JP: *Platelets: Physiology and Pathology.* New York, Stratton Inter-Continental Medical Book Corp, 1977.
40. O'Neil BP, Mann JD: Aspirin prophylaxis in migraine. *Lancet* 2:1179–1181, 1979.
41. Barcia-Marino G: El tratamiento de la Jaqueca y otras defaleas con dipiridamol. *Med Clin* 55:195–200, 1970.
42. Ostfeld AM: A study of migraine pharmacotherapy. *Am J Med Sci* 241:192–198, 1961.
43. Sutherland JM, Eadie, MJ: The drug therapy of migraine. *Med J Aust* 2:740–742, 1961.
44. Graham JR: *Treatment of Migraine.* Boston, Little, Brown, 1955.
45. Diamond S, Medina JL: Isometheptene: A non-ergot drug in the treatment of migraine. *Headache* 15:211–213, 1975.

Chapter 4
Update: Biofeedback in the Treatment of Vascular Headache

SEYMOUR DIAMOND, M.D.
JUDI DIAMOND-FALK
JOHN W. LARGEN, JR., Ph.D.

In this report we examine the effect of various modalities of biofeedback training on different types of vascular headaches. Clinical application of biofeedback technology requires that the physiological and psychological changes be measured reliably, that biofeedback training be transferred from the laboratory to the patient's natural habitat (home, school, office), that changes be of sufficient magnitude to be clinically useful, and that they be durable. Finally, the induced changes should be relatively free of serious side effects.

Clinical and experimental research has been directed toward assessing the effectiveness of several modalities of biofeedback training. These include thermal feedback, electromyographic (EMG) feedback, alpha feedback, galvanic skin response (GSR), and feedback designed to produce vasoconstriction of the temporal artery.

Vascular headaches can be divided into the following types: migraine (classical and nonclassical), cluster, unilateral facial pain, ophthalmoplegic migraine, hemiplegic migraine, toxic, and hypertensive. Most biofeedback research, however, has been directed toward migraine and cluster headaches.

REVIEW OF RESEARCH

Wolff [1] first documented that during the headache phase itself, pulsation of the temporal artery is increased. In his neurogenic theory of migraine headache he proposed that vasodilation of cerebral circulation takes place after a threat to adequate blood supply to the brain has occurred. If the rebound cerebrovascular dilation is great enough, the extracranial arteries will dilate and release a number of vasoactive substances with production of edema and a lowering of pain threshold.

This is consistent with a serendipitous finding at the Menninger Foundation. A subject who aborted her headache while participating in an experiment also noted that she had an increase in hand temperature. This led to further research at the Menninger Foundation in which Sargent et al. [2–4] experimented with autogenic feedback training. Their combination of thermal feedback with autogenic training involved simultaneous management of mental and somatic functions. "Passive concentration" was used to induce specific physiological changes, i.e., hand warmth, by focusing on visual, auditory, and somatic imagery. Each training session consisted of practicing two sets of autogenic phrases. The first set taught subjects passive concentration and relaxation of the entire body; the second set involved focusing on achieving warm hands. This was followed by the visualization of images while using a temperature trainer. These exercises were accompanied by daily practice and accurate record-keeping at home. In the earlier Menninger studies, feedback consisted of a measurement of the difference between forehead and finger temperature. It was later found, however, that the same results could be accomplished by using the finger as the only feedback site. The major change in temperature was found to occur in the hands rather than in the forehead, and most subjects reported that a positive response was primarily associated with the feeling of change in the hands rather than in the forehead.

Subjects were first seen weekly until they consistently showed a positive response. The training phase was later limited to one month, since it was found that most subjects were able to learn the techniques rapidly. Follow-up sessions were every one to three months, with the follow-up period lasting at least a year. Baseline data, consisting of headache intensity and the use of medication, were collected for the month before subjects began training. In the first pilot study, 63 percent of the 20 migraine sufferers were evaluated as improved, and in the second pilot study, 74 percent of the 63 migraine sufferers improved. The criteria for improvement were based on a decrease in headache severity, and the type and dose of analgesic used. In the follow-up evaluation, Solbach and Sargent [5] found that 55 subjects (74 percent of those who had completed 270 days of training and follow-up sessions) had a 26 percent or greater reduction of headache activity which lasted for at least two years after the study was concluded.

Another Menninger Foundation study conducted by Pearse et al. [6] was designed to reduce the duration of training. Subjects were given intensive autogenic biofeedback training for five days. Records were kept of frequency, severity, and duration of headaches, degree of disability, and medications used. Twenty-one patients were studied, 11 with migraine headaches and 10 with combination migraine and tension headaches. The results showed the five-day program to be as beneficial as the longer six-week program.

Peper and Grossman [7] trained two children with migraine headaches in thermal biofeedback and autogenic techniques. Both children learned very rapidly and were able to use what they had learned in their daily lives. Werder [8] studied four childhood migraine sufferers between the ages of 10 and 17 who were seen at the Menninger Foundation Headache Clinic. The subjects were taught to increase hand temperature and relaxation, using body awareness exercises, breathing techniques, and autogenic phrases. All four subjects learned the self-regulation of hand temperature easily. It appears that the relaxation response was easy to elicit in children, perhaps due to their lack of skepticism about the possibility of autonomic control. Lynch et al. [9] found in two experiments that four children were able to acquire instrumental control over skin temperature with visual feedback.

Russ et al. [10] conducted a follow-up study to evaluate physiological values and self-reported headache intensity nine months after the end of treatment with 16 of 50 patients who were treated with biofeedback. Patients with migraine headaches had received sessions in autogenic training in which they focused on producing sensations of heaviness and warmth in the limbs. They also received hand temperature feedback. Additionally, to rule out the possibility of experimenter effects, the follow-up examination was performed by an individual uninvolved with the treatment. Subjects noted a decline (nonsignificant) in headache activity, decreased medication usage, and subjective improvement of headache status since the end of treatment.

Drury et al. [11] used a multiple-baseline design to examine the effectiveness of a biofeedback procedure in treatment of four migraine headache patients. After baseline data were collected, the treatment consisted of cognitive preparation, modified relaxation training, autogenic phrases, finger temperature feedback, and self-charting of headaches and medication use. A positive relationship between the treatment, rated headache intensity, and recorded medication usage was found.

Mitch et al. [12] used a 12-week treatment program with autogenic phrases and continuous temperature feedback training in treating migraine. Results were evaluated based on changes in headache duration, frequency, intensity, and medications in comparison to a six-month baseline period. Eleven subjects showed improvement, with eight having "good or excellent" results and three having "fair or average" improvement. Those who improved the most were characterized as having typical migraine, while the others also had daily tension headaches and high levels of medication, did not learn the technique, or did not complete the program.

Other investigators have also used thermal feedback techniques but have omitted autogenic phrases in treating vascular headaches. Wickramasekera [13] first treated two patients with EMG feedback training without success. Later, when hand temperature training was employed, duration and intensity of headaches diminished as hand-warming skills improved. Turin and Johnson [14] trained seven subjects in the use of imagery and self-verbalization to increase peripheral temperature, rather than using autogenic phrases. They found significant decreases on all three indexes of migraine activity: numbers of headaches, headache pills, and hours of headache pain each week. They concluded that finger temperature warming, without autogenic training, is effective in reducing migraine activity, independent of suggestion effects. Additionally, to control for placebo-expectancy effects, Turin and Johnson trained their subjects in thermal cooling as well as in warming techniques. Headache activity decreased with finger warming while remaining the same or increasing with cooling, despite the subjects' positive therapeutic expectations. It was concluded that the positive effect of warming over cooling argued against attributing the positive results to relaxation or time-out rather than to the temperature training itself.

Kewman and Roberts [15] studied 34 migraine sufferers in a double-blind experiment. One experimental group was trained to raise finger temperature, one group to lower finger temperature, and a control group did not receive any finger temperature training but kept records of their migraine activity for a 21-week period—six weeks pretraining, nine weeks of training, and six weeks posttraining. Research assistants were blind to hypothesis, experimental variables, and the group to which each subject was assigned. No significant differences were found between the three groups for any of the dependent measures. All three groups showed significant improvement in the amount of impairment per headache, the number of headache symptoms, and the type and amount of medication taken. The authors concluded that nonspecific factors are as powerful as those due to temperature training. Mullinix et al. [16] had similar findings after studying 12 migraine headache patients randomly assigned to either a treatment or control group. Patients were trained in six 30-minute sessions in handwarming biofeedback and were instructed to practice twice a day at home without feedback and whenever a headache occurred. The control group had the same training and instructions but received a false feedback signal that was controlled by the investigator and was independent of any actual hand temperature change. The false signal was in a positive direction suggesting an increase in hand temperature. Patients kept a careful headache record for a minimum of five weeks prior to, during, and three months after training. The true biofeedback group obtained consistently higher hand temperatures. Medication intake remained the same or decreased for both groups, showing similar improvement in their headaches. Mullinix et al. conclude that the results suggest that biofeedback techniques are useful in treating migraine headaches, but the effect is not correlated with skin temperature changes. They hypothesize that expectation and suggestion may be the critical factors.

In a 1920s study, Hadfield [17] demonstrated that it is possible to change the temperature of the skin dramatically by direct suggestion. Much research since that time has been directed toward discovering the mechanisms underlying temperature control and factors that influence the learning of such control. Taub and Emurian [18] taught 21 subjects to increase and decrease hand temperature by using biofeedback. After lengthy stabilization periods, subjects received four sessions of operant shaping of small variations in skin temperature by means of a visual information display. Individuals varied widely in their ability to achieve self-regulatory control of skin temperature. Some were capable of only slight control, while approximately a third demonstrated changes of considerable magnitude (8–15 degrees within 15 minutes). Retention over a several month period was good. Taub furthermore concluded that feedback from a single body site may involve a different mechanism than temperature feedback with autogenic phrases, as the latter involves changes in many physiological parameters over the entire body. Asterita and Fedorchak [19] found that a sampling of eight normal volunteers was able to significantly increase the surface temperature of their dominant hand, with small increases also in other peripheral body sites such as the right wrist, arm, and ankle, as well as the left palm and wrist. The forehead region showed no significant temperature change. To make sure that observed temperature changes are the result of self-regulation and are under voluntary control, Kaplan and Crawford [20] used a technique they call target training. After achieving some success with temperature training, the client selects a target temperature as a goal and attempts to raise his temperature to that point and no higher. The researchers believe that this may be more successful than attempting to teach bidirectional control, as not all patients can accomplish this.

Taub and Emurian [21] have suggested that the control of skin temperature is due to a direct effect on volume blood flow and is not the result of muscular activity since: subjects' EMG recordings were not found to be correlated with observed temperature changes; those who practiced muscular contractions showed only small changes in skin temperature; and temperature regulation was limited to a precise locus, not a diffuse one.

Taub and Emurian [21] have reported than none of the Minnesota Multiphasic Personality Inventory scales correlate with the ability to alter skin temperature. Thompson [22], however, found the Spielberger State-Trait Anxiety Inventory and the Barratt Impulsiveness Scales to be somewhat predictive of success in normal subjects. Subjects who were highly anxious showed significantly larger initial increases in skin temperature than did subjects with low scores in anxiety. The subjects who displayed the most learning were those with high impulsivity scores and low anxiety scores. Werbach and Sandweiss [23] found that migraine patients had significantly lower finger temperatures prior to relaxation training and tended to decrease their finger temperature during their first biofeedback session more than patients suffering from other medical problems.

Roberts et al. [24] proposed that subjects could learn to voluntarily control the skin temperature of one hand relative to the other. They studied six subjects who had received extensive hypnotic training prior to the experiment. It was found that some individuals were capable of achieving a high degree of voluntary control over the autonomic processes involved in peripheral skin temperature regulation; however, there were significant individual differences in ability to learn, rate of learning, and magnitude of control that could be achieved. The variables of hypnosis and auditory feedback were confounded in the study, so it is not known whether hypnosis is a necessary adjunct to the learning process.

Roberts et al. [25] compared seven subjects who scored high in hypnotic susceptibility and absorption with seven low-scoring subjects who were trained to produce differences in skin temperatures in one hand relative to the other. They concluded from their study that some subjects can learn skin temperature control if they are provided with sufficient training and are sufficiently motivated. They found that there were significant individual differences in learning ability and that hypnotic susceptibility was not a necessity for learning. They proposed that psychophysiological variables such as autonomic responsivity, interpersonal variables such as attitude toward and relationship to the experimenter, and attitudinal and motivational variables are more likely to account for differences in learning.

Maslach et al. [26] tried to demonstrate in their study that three hypnotic subjects would be able to achieve simultaneous alteration of skin temperature in opposite directions in their two hands, while six waking control subjects would not. It was found that all of the hypnotic subjects were able to produce significant bilateral skin temperature changes, while none of the waking control subjects could master such control. The researchers argued that hypnosis provides a set of training conditions that permits a greater than normal degree of generalized relaxation, a removal of distraction stimuli, and enhanced concentration on a given relevant dimension. However, when Turin [27] compared three techniques to train subjects in finger temperature control—biofeedback, hypnosis, and a combination of the two—no differences were found between the types of training.

Keefe [28] trained eight subjects in either raising or lowering finger temperature as compared with forehead temperature. They were successfully conditioned to change their skin temperature with the use of feedback and response-specific instructions and without the use of autogenic phrases or hypnotic suggestions. Leeb et at. [29] investigated the effects of instructional sets—positive, negative, or neutral—on 15 subjects' ability to acquire hand temperature control. A significant influence was found, suggesting that the instructional set communicated by the experimenter may determine the individual's ability to learn autogenic biofeedback hand temperature training. However, Thompson [30] compared training with nontraining in autogenic finger temperature biofeedback, and positive with neutral therapeutic expectancy, and found that all four groups improved.

Mathew et al. [31] randomly assigned 12 normal subjects to either a hand-warming or a hand-cooling biofeedback group to investigate the effect of hand warming (or cooling) on intracerebral circulation. Following an extensive five-week training period in temperature biofeedback, the subjects were given two consecutive measures of noninvasive regional cerebral blood flow, using the ^{133}Xenon inhalation technique. One measure of regional cerebral blood flow was taken during a relaxed condition and a second measure while subjects were actively trying to change their hand skin temperature in the trained direction with biofeedback. The mean cerebral blood flow of both the warming and cooling groups tended to remain the same or shift in similar directions, even though the subjects were manipulating their skin temperatures in opposite directions. The results suggest that the therapeutic gains described in migraine therapy may be due not to a factor specific to temperature biofeedback but possibly to some more general factor, such as relaxation or passive concentration, or to the demand characteristics of the situation. However, Largen et al. [32] then conducted a similar experiment with 13 migraine patients and found that, as the hand-warming and hand-cooling groups regulated their hand skin temperature in opposite directions, cerebral blood flow changes of the two groups were significantly different. Skin temperature changes were found to be related to cerebral blood flow. In comparison to normal volunteers, migraine sufferers had greater cerebral vasomotor reactivity. Cerebral blood flow during skin temperature self-regulation differed greatly between migraine headache sufferers and normal volunteers. Eighty-three percent of the hand-warming patients showed large decreases in headache frequency, while 80 percent of the hand-cooling group showed an increase. This supports the theory that specific temperature factors are responsible for the effectiveness of temperature biofeedback rather than just relaxation or placebo-expectancy effects.

Sovak et al. [33] studied the effects of vasodilation in the hands resulting from either induced heat or feedback training on the carotid vasculature. The subjects, five normal and 12 migraine sufferers, were taught a relaxation technique with autogenic phrases involving the adaptation-relaxation reflex. The blood vessels in the hand and arm dilate, which is associated with reduced blood flow in the temporal arteries. After the subjects had mastered the hand-warming technique, the experiment was conducted. Finger temperature was recorded as well as pulse volumes of the finger and the frontotemporal region by reflectance photoplethysmography. Eight of the ten migraineurs who learned the hand-warming technique were evaluated as clinically improved. With volitional feedback, the pulse volume increased in the finger and decreased in the frontotemporal region in improved migraineurs and normals. With heat, the normals and unimproved migraineurs showed an increase in the frontotemporal regions, while there was a decrease with the improved migraineurs.

Another modality of biofeedback, involving the operant conditioning of vasoconstriction of the extracranial artery, has been used by various investigators. The treatment model derives from the classical migraine theory of Wolff, according to which the pain associated with migraine is primarily the result of vasodilation of branches of the external carotid artery. Koppman et al. [34] had ten migraine patients attempt to modify their temporal artery diameter by using biofeedback techniques. Through the use of a reflectance photoplethysmometer, seven subjects were able

UPDATE: BIOFEEDBACK IN TREATMENT 45

to learn dilation-constriction sequences with considerable proficiency in two to four weeks with two or three sessions per week. Savill and Koppman [35] trained six nonmigrainous subjects to develop control over the blood volume pulse amplitude in either the temporal artery or the finger. Simultaneously, blood volume pulse was recorded at both locations and skin temperature was recorded on the finger that held a photoplethysmometer. They found that temporal artery blood volume pulse measures are as simple to obtain as finger skin temperature measures.

Friar and Beatty [36] investigated the operant training of nine experimental subjects taught to vasoconstrict the extracranial arteries and nine control group subjects taught vasoconstriction of the hand, an irrelevant site. All of the subjects suffered from severe and frequent migraine headaches. Arterial pulse waves were recorded from the surface of the skin with pressure plethysmographs during eight training sessions. The experimental group, which demonstrated control of the affected extracranial arteries, showed a reduction on all indices of migraine headache except intensity, and in all categories of medication, while the control group showed no significant improvement in symptomatology.

Zamani [37] also treated migraine patients with operant conditioning of vasoconstriction of the extracranial temporal artery or deep muscle relaxation. The biofeedback group changed significantly in average number of hours of headache per week, and average length of each headache. The relaxation group showed no significant decrease of any of the variables.

Bild [38] studied 19 migraineurs trained in cephalic vasomotor response feedback (CVMR) or frontalis EMG feedback and a waiting list control group. Both types of feedback were found to reduce the duration of the migraine headaches, with CVMR feedback having a greater effect and also reducing medication intake. Feuerstein and Adams [39] investigated the effect of cephalic vasomotor response and frontalis electromyographic feedback on control of temporal arterial vasoconstriction and frontalis muscle activity in migraine and muscle contraction headache patients, using a single-subject multiple-baseline design. Both migraine and muscle contraction patients received six EMG and six CVMR feedback training sessions in a counterbalanced sequence. Each patient completed a daily headache form that included ratings of frequency, duration, and intensity, recorded during the baseline, feedback, and follow-up conditions. The changes in headache activity were significant for all but one patient; however, consistent reductions in frequency and duration of headaches were observed in this patient. The greatest reduction in headache activity occurred when feedback was directed at the relevant pain mechanism.

Price and Tursky [40] studied 40 migraine sufferers and 40 controls assigned to one of four treatments: feedback, false feedback, relaxation tape, and a neutral tape control. Four physiological measures—digital blood volume and pulse volume, cephalic blood volume and pulse volume —were monitored while the subjects were instructed to try to increase their hand temperature. The results showed differences between migraine sufferers and normals in digital vascular responses, with migraine subjects less able than normals to produce vasodilation. Even greater differences between migraine subjects and normals were found for temporal artery blood volume changes. Biofeedback produced greater digital vasodilation than did relaxation produced by listening to an irrelevant tape recording; however, there was no statistically significant advantage of biofeedback over a false-feedback treatment or a relaxation treatment. These results can be interpreted in two ways: digital vasodilation can be produced by any treatment that seems valid to a subject, or any active treatment aimed at increasing vasodilation is more effective than nontreatment. The correlation found between digital and temporal blood volume changes does not support the hypothesis that increasing blood volume in the hand results in decreases in the head. The authors conclude that increased blood flow to the hands is most likely a component of general relaxation.

Electromyographic feedback involves the monitoring of muscle tension. Very little research has been conducted on the use of electromyographic feedback alone in the treatment of vascular headaches. Bakal and Kaganov [41] studied 10 patients, five suffering from muscle contraction headaches and five migraineurs. They completed 15 frontalis EMG biofeedback training sessions and also received deep-muscle relaxation training. They were encouraged to practice both at home. The patients kept headache records during biofeedback training and both groups showed a significant decrease in headache scores. Additionally, migraine patients were found to have significantly higher frontalis EMG activity than muscle contraction headache patients, both during a headache attack and when headache-free.

Other types of relaxation therapy and autogenic training have also been examined. Mitchell [42] and Mitchell and Mitchell [43], in conducting four controlled studies of migraine headaches, compared "combined desensitization," involving relaxation training, desensitization, and assertive therapy, with each form of therapy alone. The combined treatment was most successful, with an average 66.8 percent reduction in the number of migraine attacks, possibly because it dealt with the environmental events surrounding migraine as well as with the migraine itself. They speculate that the assertive training may have been the most important variable, since migraine may result from inhibiting the expression of emotion or an inability to cope with stress. In a six-year investigation, Hay and Madders [44] treated patients referred for relaxation therapy who had two or more disabling migraines in a month and were resistant to pharmacological treatments. Of these, 69 patients showed a decrease in severity, frequency, or duration of attacks, 25 showed no change, and four experienced a worsening of their headaches.

Blanchard et al. [45] studied 30 migraine patients by randomly assigning them to three treatment groups after a four-week baseline period. One group used finger temperature biofeedback, autogenic training, and home practice; another used progressive relaxation training and home practice; and the third was a waiting list control group. Blanchard et al. found that both the relaxation group and the biofeedback group improved significantly on total headache activity, duration of headaches, peak headache intensity, and analgesic medication usage, while the control group did not. All three groups showed significant decreases in headache frequency. The biofeedback group and the relaxation group did not differ on any dependent measure. Silver et al. [46] then studied one year after treatment 18 of 26 subjects who had learned either temperature biofeedback or progressive relaxation techniques. They evaluated the long-term effectiveness of the two types of treatment on migraine headaches. The subjects completed a headache questionnaire and kept headache data, including medicine consumption and headache activity. The two groups did not differ on any measure except the medication index, with the relaxation training group consuming less medication. Both groups had maintained their therapeutic gains at three-month and one-year follow-ups, although they did not continue with regular practice. Thus, no differential efficacy was determined between temperature biofeedback or progressive relaxation for the treatment of migraine.

Luthe and Schultz [47] found that a majority of patients who received autogenic therapy showed a decrease in frequency and intensity of migraine attacks. Autogenic training involves the simultaneous regulation of mental and somatic functions. The desired somatic responses are evoked by passive concentration on phrases, with patients first attempting to bring under control heaviness in the limbs and warmth in the extremities.

Research has been developed that combines both thermal and electromyographic feedback. Fahrion [48] noted that hand temperature decreases during stress and increases with relaxation, with vasoconstriction during stress being part of an adaptive biological pattern that prepares the body for flight by moving the blood from the periphery and into the deep muscles, the myocardium, and the head. In comparing the effects of stress and relaxation on finger temperature response, Baudewyns [49] also found that finger temperature decreased under stress conditions and increased under relaxation conditions. Many investigators using thermal feedback alone have commenced with relaxation training. Taub [18] has emphasized the influential role of emotional state on hand temperature, explaining that the laboratory situation is a tense one and anxiety tends to decrease the temperature of the extremities. When allowed time to adjust to the situation, subjects who were tense begin to relax and hand temperature consequently increases. Taub warns against confusing the effects of general relaxation with those of specific training. This can occur by starting a training session before the initial relaxation process is completed.

It is felt that relaxation facilitates the ability to learn thermal feedback control. Pearse et al. [6] found that the ability to regularly reach a good degree of relaxation was vital in learning voluntary control of hand warmth. Culver and Hauri [unpublished, 1972] have proposed that since learning to control vasomotor tone in the hands is easier when patients are in a relaxed state, skin temperature training would be most efficiently accomplished when preceded by EMG skeletal muscle training. Scott and Timmons [50] found that a tense subject has low finger temperature and high EMG tension; as he relaxes, finger temperature increases because relaxed muscles consume less energy and generate less heat. If a subject begins a session already very relaxed, finger temperature may not change. With initial relaxation, the reservoir of excess heat is dissipated, leading to an increase in finger temperature followed by skin cooling. The investigators feel that generally a reduction of stress through relaxation is also involved. EMG biofeedback also often serves as a good "ice-breaker" for later temperature feedback. Some propose that EMG feedback is easier to learn, shows quicker results, and, perhaps most importantly, leaves the subject with a sense of self-esteem and self-control.

Many investigators have used both thermal and electromyographic feedback modalities for treating vascular headaches. Diamond et al. [unpublished, 1975] studied the response of 382 patients to different modalities of biofeedback therapy. Patients in training practiced progressive relaxation exercises followed by EMG training, and/or hand temperature control training with autogenic phrases. The training period consisted of two office sessions per week for one month, or a more intensified two-week training period for 36 out-of-town patients, with home practice of hand-warming techniques and relaxation. All patients received follow-up training sessions every two months. Headache and medication records were kept. Responses to treatment were rated as follows: good—a consistent decrease in the number and severity of headaches; fair—a decrease in either frequency or severity of headaches; no response—a failure to respond to treatment. For training, 103 patients received only EMG feedback, 45 patients received only hand temperature feedback, and 234 patients received a combination of both hand temperature and EMG feedback. The investigators found that with EMG feedback alone administered to ten migraine patients, two showed a good response and eight a negative response; of the 62 mixed migraine and muscle-contraction headache patients, 23 had a good, two a fair, and 37 a negative response. When hand temperature feedback alone was administered to 20 migraine patients, 17 had a good response and three a negative response, while the 25 mixed muscle-contraction and migraine headache patients showed eight good and 17 negative responses. The responses of those 53 migraine patients receiving a combination of EMG and temperature feedback were 38 good, four fair, and 11 negative, while for the 167 mixed muscle-contraction and migraine headache patients there were 75 good, 11 fair, and 81 negative responses. The results indicated that patients with migraine headaches responded well to either hand temperature feedback, with 85 percent of patients improving, or to the combination of EMG and hand temperature feedback, with 79 percent improving. No significant effects were noted with any of the three techniques in the mixed muscle-contraction and migraine headache patients; however, the combination of both temperature and EMG feedback did result in an improvement in about 50 percent of the patients.

Diamond and Franklin [51] compared 36 headache patients in an intensive training program with 57 patients receiving the routine training. The intensive program consisted of two temperature and EMG feedback sessions per day for 12 days and a one-month follow-up session. The routine training involved two sessions weekly for a four-week period and then a gradual weaning to more infrequent sessions as response to therapy indicated. Response to treatment was rated as good, fair, or no response. Results for the 36 intensive therapy patients were 18 good, one fair, and 17 negative responses; the results for those in routine therapy were 38 good, three fair, and 16 negative responses. Among patients receiving intensive training, there was a 90 percent success rate in straight vascular headaches, with only a 41 percent success rate in mixed vascular and muscle-contraction headache patients. In the routine group, 76 percent of the vascular patients and 68 percent of the patients with mixed diagnosis were successful. The differences were not found to be significant between intensive and routine biofeedback therapy. A contrast was seen between patients' success during training and failure in follow-up visits, as patients often returned to the clinic with reports of no headache change and showed decreasing abilities on the temperature trainer. The major problem was found to be incorporating the intensive training into everyday life.

Medina et al. [52] studied 27 patients with migraine or mixed migraine and muscle-contraction headaches who had been trained in EMG and skin temperature control at least six months earlier. All patients kept complete records of the number and intensity of headaches and the amount of abortive medications taken, which were compared with the last two months prior to biofeedback training. Significant reductions on all three measures were noted in 13 of the 27 patients. Nine of the 14 with migraine headaches (64 percent) were improved, while only four of 13 mixed migraine and muscle-contraction headache sufferers improved.

Diamond and Franklin [53] used autogenic training with both electromyographic and temperature feedback in treating 32 children with migraine headaches. The importance of daily home practice was stressed and records of home sessions were kept. Twenty-six children had good results, with decreases in both the frequency and severity of migraine headaches; three showed fair results, decreasing either frequency or severity; two showed no response; and one patient was lost to follow-up.

Diamond et al. [54] conducted a five-year retrospective study to examine the long-term effects of biofeedback training on headache problems. The clinic sessions were composed of three stages: skin temperature feedback with autogenic training, muscle-relaxation exercises, and electromyographic feedback. The home sessions included muscle-relaxation exercises and temperature feedback. Questionnaires were mailed to all patients who had completed training and these self-report assessment scores were evaluated with a chi-square design. It was found that biofeedback training was significantly more effective, decreased more headache pain, had training effects last a longer time, and taught greater relaxation techniques for younger patients, female patients, and those patients with no past drug habituation problem. The longer the time since training, the less effective biofeedback was found to be. A relationship was seen between the effectiveness of biofeedback training and the type of headache. Patients with vascular headaches were most helped; those with mixed vascular and muscle-contraction headaches were next; the least affected were patients with muscle-contraction headaches.

Fried et al. [55] used a combination of biofeedback-mediated electromyographical relaxation and autogenic feedback training to assist six patients suffering from migraine, tension, or mixed vascular-tension headaches. Patients kept data sheets monitoring the frequency and duration of headaches two weeks before starting treatment and over the treatment period, which extended, according to each patient's needs, from one month to a year. EMG and autogenic phrases to aid in practicing relaxation were administered for the first two weeks of training and then temperature trainers and audiotapes were introduced. Three patients showed little or questionable improvement, while three showed greater than 75 percent improvement based on severity of headaches, drug potency, and number of drugs used to control the headache pain. Fried et al. concluded that patients are often lacking the necessary motivation to profit from psychological intervention and that home practice is critical to success in treatment.

Hartje and Diver [56] studied the assumption that there is extensive vasoconstriction in the hands as a result of sympathetic overactivation before the onset of a migraine headache. Fourteen subjects were trained in EMG and thermal feedback techniques. Only three migraine sufferers were analyzed for a decrease in hand temperature preceding an increase in headache severity. The investigators found that some migraine sufferers may be able to reliably predict the onset or worsening of a migraine headache by simply monitoring hand temperature.

Aside from the beneficial effects of relaxation on thermal feedback control, relaxation also plays a major role in alleviating the vascular headache itself. Pozniak-Patewicz [57] found that during migraine headaches there is a marked muscle spasm in the head and neck muscles that, in some instances, can be even more prominent than the muscle tension noted in muscle-contraction headaches. Muscle tension not only has a role in initiating the vascular headache but also increases its severity. Stress is one of the many factors that may precipitate migraine attacks. Thus, some investigators have combined temperature feedback, electromyographic feedback, and various other relaxation techniques in treating vascular headaches. Beasley [58] studied 37 migraine sufferers, comparing those receiving relaxation exercises and autogenic suggestion with finger temperature biofeedback with those receiving only finger temperature biofeedback, relaxation exercises with autogenic suggestions alone, or a nontreatment control group. It was found that only the biofeedback group combined with relaxation exercises and autogenic suggestions benefited.

Adler and Adler [59] studied headache patients who had terminated treatment three and a half to five years earlier. We looked at only those with vascular headaches—22 migraine, 12 mixed migraine and tension headache, and five cluster headache patients. Patients were given temperature feedback training after an initial period of EMG feedback. They also received concomitant psychotherapy. The success rate for migraine was 81 percent, for mixed headache 60 percent, and for cluster headache 60 percent. The authors believe that the essential factor in the maintained improvement was the therapeutic interweaving of both psychologic and physiologic facets of headache management. They believe that the patients' new-found ability to relax is often as important to them as the relief from headache since it gives them a new way to deal with stress.

Boller and Flom [60] have proposed that common migraine, without the prodromata associated with classical migraine, is less available to modification via single-modality biofeedback training. They found that a 12-week program combining autogenic training, thermal feedback, and, occasionally, EMG feedback, patient education, and counseling provides a reasonable approach to moderating the common migraine. Their program relied heavily on consistent practice of relaxation techniques and cognitive integration of the environmental stressors that trigger headaches.

Werbach and Sandweiss [61] retrospectively studied 45 migraine headache sufferers. Patients were told that the goal of the program was to assist them in learning a "relaxation response" that was thought to be correlated with decreased migraine activity. Measurements of digital finger temperature, palmar skin conductance, and frontalis EMG were made before and after each session, with biofeedback being continuously provided from one of the three physiologic variables. Other relaxation procedures were also introduced, including abdominal breathing techniques, a modification of Jacobson's progressive muscle relaxation, meditative mantras, and autogenic phrases. Criteria for improvement included reduction in headache frequency or intensity, smaller amounts of medication needed for pain relief, or achievement of an ability to abort migraines. Of the 37 patients who completed 10 training sessions, 73 percent were rated improved, with younger patients improving the most. There was a total lack of correlation between temperature gain scores across sessions and treatment outcome; the ability to warm hands was not found to be related to a reduction in migraine activity.

Weinstock [62] studied seven patients who suffered from either tension or migraine headaches. Patients practiced self-induced hypnotic relaxation in the first session, followed by EMG biofeedback in the remaining sessions. Thermal feedback was then started for the following four to ten sessions, depending on the patient's progress. All seven patients were functioning without headaches four months or more after treatment.

Few researchers have used alpha feedback in the treatment of vascular headaches. Cannon and Sternbach [63] found that a subject who received prolonged alpha training was able to delay the onset of migraine headaches but could not modify the pain once the headache had begun. Melzack and Perry [64] believe that four variables contribute to pain relief in the alpha feedback training procedure: distraction of attention, suggestion, relaxation, and the development of a sense of control over pain, thereby lessening the level of perceived pain. The relaxation that accompanies the "alpha state" can produce a decrease in sensory outputs. Although they did not study vascular headaches specifically, Melzack and Perry found that alpha feedback training methods appear to provide an effective technique for the self-regulation of pain but must be accompanied by hypnotic training, placebo effects, and progressive relaxation techniques. Kasanof [65], however, concluded that self-control of EEG signals in the alpha range has little, if any, clinical application, and that there is no controlled experimental evidence that the ability to turn alpha waves on and off has any therapeutic value. He believes there is evidence that many "alpha trainers" do not really detect alpha waves but merely respond to secondary effects of general relaxation.

Two other groups of investigators have studied alpha feedback in comparing various modalities of biofeedback and their effect on migraine headaches. Andreychuck and Skriver [66] studied three treatment procedures with 33 migraine headache sufferers—biofeedback training for hand warming, biofeedback training for alpha enhancement, and training for self-hypnosis. A Headache Index was compiled for six weeks prior to the treatment program and the last five weeks of treatment. The Hypnotic Induction Profile was used to obtain hypnotic susceptibility scores for each subject. The three different treatment groups all showed significant reductions of headaches, and there were no significant differences in improvement among the treatment groups. The temperature biofeedback group did show a higher percentage improvement rate than either the alpha biofeedback group or the self-hypnosis group, although the results were not statistically significant. The highly hypnotizable subjects showed significant reductions in headaches when compared with the low hypnotizable subjects. However, each of the treatments also focused considerably on relaxation, and this may have been the crucial variable involved. Cohen et al. [67] studied 45 migraine patients who received three modalities of biofeedback training. Patients were treated with temperature feedback, muscle relaxation, or EEG for an eight-week training period of three sessions per week. Temperature and EMG self-regulation were found to be more therapeutic than EEG alpha feedback in treating migraine.

Two studies have been conducted that compare temperature biofeedback and hypnosis. Graham [68] studied 30 migraineurs who were susceptible to hypnosis. They were divided into three groups; each group received either hypnosis, finger temperature feedback, or a combination of hypnosis and finger temperature feedback. No differences were found among the groups; all improved on all migraine variables. Crosson et al.

[69] studied seven migrainous subjects who were divided into two groups. One group listened to a self-hypnosis tape, practiced autogenic suggestion phrases, and received hand temperature biofeedback, while the other group received no hypnosis and only the autogenic biofeedback training. The results suggested that hypnosis treatment led to physiological changes similar to those obtained with biofeedback.

No research is available concerning galvanic skin response in the treatment of vascular headaches.

RESULTS OF RESEARCH

The results of numerous studies have indicated that thermal feedback, either in conjunction with autogenic training or alone, is beneficial in treating vascular headaches. The Sargent group's [2–4] results have indicated that 60 to 75 percent of patients who completed autogenic feedback training improved their migraine headaches. However, many researchers have criticized the findings for various reasons. Taub [70] found many factors that prevent unambiguous interpretation of the Menninger studies: there were no data on temperature self-regulation performance, the number who succeeded in learning the task or the extent of control achieved. The conditions of training and testing were not held constant, the assessment of headache symptoms were unstandardized, and there were no controls for placebo effects. Price [71] found other elements missing from the research. Pretreatment baseline data were not available for most of the participants. There was no statistical treatment of the data, only the judgment of improvement by three evaluators, and no control groups of any kind (i.e., attention placebo, false feedback, autogenic training without feedback) were used. Blanchard and Young [72] criticized the work of the Menninger group, finding the presentation of the results to be poor. Of 75 patients in the total sample, adequate data for clinical ratings were available for only 62, of which an unspecified number were migraine sufferers; 74 percent of the latter group were rated as improved. Pretraining data were available for only 32 migraine patients. There was reportedly "poor agreement" between evaluators on improvement; of 32 patients, 29 were rated improved by one evaluator, 26 by another evaluator, and 22 by the third evaluator. Blanchard and Young believe that no substantive conclusions on the therapeutic efficacy of hand warming can be drawn for three reasons: little information on results is given and post-treatment results are not statistically significant, the treatment package itself is a combination of several factors—suggestion, relaxation training, and biofeedback training, and there were no placebo or no-treatment control groups provided. Jessup et al. [73] believe that the most encouraging results for temperature training biofeedback appear in uncontrolled studies. They concluded that decreases in migraine symptoms are apparently due to nonspecific factors with finger temperature change irrelevant to symptom reduction.

Fahrion [48], however, has argued that the various studies support the hypothesis that biofeedback is causally related to a reduction of migraine and is not effective simply because it mobilizes placebo-suggestion factors, since placebo medications typically produce improvements in only 5 to 25 percent of patients tested, not the 70 to 80 percent found improved in many biofeedback studies. Wickramasekera [13] also did not interpret his results as a placebo response because the two patients treated had been affected by migraine headaches for many years, during which time they tried many other types of treatment without success. However, Miller [74] believes that the failure of past treatments does not negate the possibility of placebo effects unless one can show that the treatments did not also result in transitory success or that the new therapy produces a long-lasting success. Turin and Johnson [14], who trained their subjects in both thermal cooling and warming techniques and observed the positive effect of warming over cooling, seem to have controlled for placebo expectancy effects.

Barber [75] concluded that at times skin temperature control may be a result of changes in arousal, while at other times it may indirectly result from localized contraction and relaxation of specific muscles or may be exerting an exercise effect on blood flow. Many researchers theorize that hand warming involves a reduction in sympathetic outflow, thus interrupting the vasomotor cycle of migraine headaches. Sargent et al. [4] hypothesized that sympathetic relaxation, not blood volume changes, is the effective agent in migraine amelioration. Stroebel and Glueck [76] supported the theory that peripheral dilatation may be accompanied by cranial dilatation. They hypothesized that hand warming may abort migraines during the prodromal stage by bringing about a generalized vasodilation that prevents the increased sympathetic outflow from reaching a rebound threshold. This implies that any method that reduces sympathetic activity may be useful as a technique for aborting migraine headaches. There has been some support for the "sympathetic outflow theory" in a combination biochemical/biofeedback study by Kentsmith et al. [77]. Norepinephrine and dopamine-beta-hydroxylase (DBH) are released into circulation in proportional amounts following stimulation of sympathetic neurons. Thus, the level of plasma DBH may serve as a rough gauge of the extent of sympathetic nervous activity. In the study, a migrainous subject was trained in the symptomatic improvement of migraine headaches through a combination of procedures that included temperature biofeedback. As a correlate of the treatment, the plasma levels of DBH were found to have decreased 32 percent, suggesting a lowering of sympathetic activity to a more normal level. Mitchell and Mitchell [43] have shown an improvement rate of 71 percent in migraine sufferers given only relaxation training. Pearse et al. [6] also found a significant positive relationship between patients' ability to relax and their headache improvement. In their study comparing thermal feedback with muscle relaxation and EEG feedback, Cohen et al. [67] found that both temperature and muscle relaxation self-regulation were more therapeutic than EEG feedback. Considering the positive effects of thermal feedback therapy and relaxation therapy investigated separately, it might follow that the combination of both thermal and electromyographic feedback would be of even greater therapeutic value in treating vascular headaches. Diamond et al. [unpublished, 1975] compared thermal feedback alone, electromyographic feedback alone, and the combination of thermal and electromyograph feedback. They found that the combination of both modalities elicited the best results.

Friar and Beatty [36] and Zamani [37] have found a beneficial therapeutic value in using feedback involving vasoconstriction of the extracranial arteries in treating migraine headaches. CVMR merits further research as a possible effective biofeedback treatment for migraine. Taub and Emurian [18] believe that there are different mechanisms involved in this technique and thermal feedback. They conclude that the hand-warming technique is effective because it involves the induction of a state of relaxation, while the vasoconstriction of arteries is constricting vessels that would otherwise cause pain due to excessive vasodilation. Jessup et al. [73] have stated that temperature feedback and temporal artery vasoconstriction are two opposing processes that have given favorable results, with temperature feedback aimed at reducing sympathetic activity and temporal artery vasoconstriction requiring increased sympathetic activity.

PRECAUTIONS, CONTRAINDICATIONS, AND OTHER INTERVENING FACTORS

Gaardner and Montgomery [78] have listed many intervening variables in assessing the suitable biofeedback candidate. Included are responses to the philosophy of treatment, ego strength, personality, motivation, nature of symptoms, the possibility that other forms of treatment should be given priority, and past experience in attempting to obtain symptom relief. Other cited variables are previous experience with other psychophysiological approaches and previous biofeedback experience, duration of treatment, placebo effects, and the experimenter. Birk [79] has noted many emotional factors in the migraine patient's personality. He found migraine sufferers to be anxious, striving, perfectionistic, order-loving, rigid. They become progressively more tense during periods of threat or conflict and show mismanagement and suppression of anger. Wolff [1] also found migraine sufferers to be tense and overconscientious. Mitchell and Mitchell [43] described the migraine personality as sensitive, worrisome, perfectionist, chronically tense, apprehensive, preoccupied by achievement and success. The migraine personality was characterized by superficial interpersonal relationships, sexual maladjustment, and obsessive preoccupation with moral and ethical issues and was more neurotic than that of nonmigraine patients. However, there are many researchers who do not believe that there is a migraine personality.

Sargent et al. [3, 4] believe that psychological factors are important in determining success or failure in learning to increase blood flow in the hands. Persons comfortable with the idea that thoughts and feelings can influence bodily processes learn faster. Also, psychologic-mindedness is helpful in learning psychosomatic self-regulation of migraine headache. Wickramasekera [80] has found a positive correlation between biofeedback skill and hypnotizability. He also noted the importance of self-discipline. The more psychologically oriented, highly motivated, and less resistant person is likely to be more receptive to biofeedback.

It is essential to make an adequate working diagnosis of the etiology of each headache. Those patients who have more than one type of headache must be distinguished. The degree of disability from the headache, the duration of the headache, and the presence of associated symptoms are other factors that must be considered. A detailed history and complete neurological examination by a physician are necessary to determine the proper biofeedback candidate. Diamond and Baltes [81] characterized vascular headaches as typically one-sided pain, with 30 to 40 percent accompanied by an aura that is usually visual. There is often a family history of such headaches. The throbbing, pulsating pain starts and builds with time and may last two to three days. Nausea and vomiting may accompany the pain. The headache may shift from side to side and occasionally be bilateral. Four times more women are afflicted than men, with the sufferers often finding relief during pregnancy or after menopause. Foods containing tyramine can evoke headaches in 30 percent of vascular headache sufferers. Patients diagnosed as having only vascular headaches are more successful with biofeedback than patients with combination headaches. More specifically, classical migraine sufferers, having an aura preceding their headaches, show better results than patients with non-classical migraine, due to the nature of the headache.

Migraine patients often have an accompanying depressive illness, indicated by a sleep disturbance. Diamond and Franklin [51] have studied headache patients with sleep disturbances who are receiving biofeedback training. There are two different types of sleep disturbances. One involves difficulty in falling asleep, primarily due to anxiety, while the other involves frequent and early awakening, primarily due to depression. Biofeedback results were not good for patients whose sleep pattern was consistent with depression. These patients may respond better in biofeedback training if they are supported with concomitant antidepressant drug therapy. Biofeedback has not been shown to be effective in treating cluster headaches, organic disease, or depression of a nonneurotic nature, but it is effective for psychoneurotic depressions.

Drug dependency is another factor reducing the chances for success with biofeedback training. Diamond and Franklin [82] after treating 119 habituated patients with a combination of thermal and electromyographic feedback, found that only 30 patients showed a good response, 18 showed a fair response, and 71 were unimproved. Fordyce et al. [83] believe that a pain habit may be present in many patients and may require alteration of reinforcement (social and physical) contingencies. Budzynski [84] found that even after learning control of muscle tension and temperature responses, some migraine patients cannot decrease their daily drug intake. They require a period of systematic desensitization to reduce anxiety before medication reduction can begin. Eventually, they can exist without medication except in extreme circumstances and will use their hand-warming techniques at the headache onset.

Children are considered good candidates for biofeedback. Sargent et al. [3, 4] found that younger persons responded more quickly to training than did older individuals, as younger persons often are less rigid and more ready to adjust to new situations. Diamond and Franklin [85] also found age to be an important factor in biofeedback therapy. The initiation of biofeedback in young children with migraine may prevent the later development of depression and drug habituation typically observed in older patients. Werbach and Sandweiss [23, 61] also found younger patients' migraine headaches improved the most after biofeedback-assisted relaxation training. However, Feuerstein et al. [86] caution against totally ruling out elderly people as biofeedback candidates, after successfully treating an elderly patient with combined muscle-contraction and migraine headaches with cephalic vasomotor and EMG feedback.

The setting and the way in which techniques are administered also play a role in the degree of success of biofeedback training. In comparing an intensive five-day training program with the longer term six-week program, Pearse et al. [6] found them to be equally beneficial. During training, Diamond and Franklin [87] also found no difference between patients participating in a two-week intensive short-term biofeedback program and those in a long-term program. A significant contrast, however, could be seen in the intensive group's success during training and failure in follow-up visits. Intensive group patients had been on a "therapeutic vacation" and had more difficulty incorporating their training into their everyday lives than patients who received the routine therapy while continuing their normal daily routine. Wickramasekera [80] stressed the need to find the optimal conditions for biofeedback training: intensive inpatient versus long-term outpatient. He believes that biofeedback training is not always reliable in the transfer of training from a clinic to a natural habitat. One possibility is to conduct the training in the natural habitat or phase the training into it. He concluded that biofeedback training may not be transferable into an inherently stressful natural habitat and may require a total treatment package.

The biofeedback administrator can affect the outcome of biofeedback training. Fahrion [48] noted great differences in the individual effectiveness of biofeedback trainers. Effective training depends on an open, warm rapport between trainer and trainee. He cautions that attempting to force the training process into a narrow, standardized form, as in a controlled study, invariably lowers the subject's ability to learn the hand-warming techniques. Taub and Emurian [18] also emphasize the large "person factor" between experimenters and subjects in training for self-regulation of skin temperature. He found that an impersonal experimenter, unconvinced of biofeedback's feasibility, was only able to train two of 22 subjects to regulate skin temperature, while a friendly, informal experimenter succeeded in training 19 of 21 subjects.

CONCLUSIONS AND FUTURE RESEARCH GOALS

Biofeedback has proven to be a worthwhile therapeutic modality in the treatment of vascular headaches, but many factors have yet to be explored. Wickramasekera [80] has listed many of the uncontrolled variables in past research on biofeedback and vascular headache, which include subject and experimenter expectations, interpersonal and relationship variables (empathy, warmth), motivation and incentives (increasing suggestibility), and baseline individual differences in readiness to learn biological self-control. Some of these factors, however, would be difficult to control in a clinical setting. Future studies must determine if there are individual differences in the ability to learn visceral control and what extracranial vascular activity accompanies temperature training in the hands. Future research into personality and psychological factors that are predictive or counterpredictive of success in applying biofeedback to vascular headaches is necessary, as is research into the effectiveness of generalization of skills learned in the laboratory to nonlaboratory situations. In order to control for placebo effects Miller [74] believes that either nontreated control groups or a long pre-treatment baseline and long post-treatment follow-up or double-blind testing is necessary. There is also the need to investigate the possibility of symptom substitution (e.g., shift from a headache problem to an ulcer problem), and to deal with the problem of volunteers not adequately representing the headache population.

Future researchers should conduct a thorough investigation into the therapeutic significance of biofeedback with types of vascular headaches other than migraine, employing better statistical analyses and methodological reporting. Future studies should also be keyed toward determining whether thermal feedback, electromyographic feedback, autogenic training, conditioning vasoconstriction of the extracranial artery, or combinations of these types of therapy are effective. It is necessary to elucidate what aspect of the therapeutic package is necessary for reducing the frequency and intensity of vascular headaches. A variety of techniques have been shown to be useful in reaching temperature control, but it is necessary to ascertain how the techniques can be combined most effectively.

REFERENCES

1. Wolff HG: *Headache and Other Head Pain*, 2nd Ed. New York, Oxford University Press, 1963.
2. Sargent JD, Green EE, Walters ED: The use of autogenic feedback training in a pilot study of migraine and tension headaches. *Headache* 12(3):120–124, 1972.
3. Sargent JD, Green EE, Walters ED: Preliminary report on the use of autogenic feedback training in the treatment of migraine and tension headaches. *Psychosom Med* 35(2):129–135, 1973.
4. Sargent JD, Green EE, Walters ED: Psychosomatic self-regulation of migraine headache, in Birk L (ed): *Biofeedback: Behavioral Medicine*. New York, Grune & Stratton, 1973, pp 55–68.
5. Solbach P, Sargent J: A follow-up evaluation of a five and one-half year migraine headache study using thermal training. Presented to Biofeedback Society of America Annual Meeting, 1977.
6. Pearse BA, Walters ED, Sargent JD: Exploratory observations of the use of an intensive autogenic biofeedback procedure in a follow-up study of out-of-town

patients having migraine and/or tension headaches. *Proceedings of Biofeedback Research Society Sixth Annual Meeting*, 1975.

7. Peper E, Grossman ER: Preliminary observation of thermal biofeedback training in children with migraine. Presented to Biofeedback Research Society Annual Meeting, 1974.

8. Werder DS: An exploratory study of childhood migraine using thermal biofeedback as a treatment alternative. *Proceedings of Biofeedback Society of America Ninth Annual Meeting*, 1978.

9. Lynch WC, Hama H, Kohn S, Miller NE: Instrumental control of peripheral vasomotor responses in children. *Psychophysiology* 13(3):219–221, 1976.

10. Russ KL, Hammer RL, Adderton M: Clinical follow-up: Treatment outcome of functional headache patients treated with biofeedback. Presented to Biofeedback Society of America Annual Meeting, 1977.

11. Drury RL, DeRisi W, Liberman R: Temperature feedback treatment for migraine headache: A controlled study. *Proceedings of Biofeedback Research Society Sixth Annual Meeting*, 1975.

12. Mitch PS, McGrady A, Iannone A: Autogenic feedback training in treatment of migraine: A clinical report. *Proceedings of Biofeedback Research Society Sixth Annual Meeting*, 1975.

13. Wickramasekera I: Temperature feedback for the control of migraine. *Behavior Therapy and Experimental Psychiatry* 4:343–345, 1973.

14. Turin A, Johnson WG: Biofeedback therapy for migraine headaches. *Arch Gen Psychiatry* 33:517–519, 1976.

15. Kewman D, Roberts AH: Skin temperature biofeedback and migraine headache: A double-blind study. *Proceedings of Biofeedback Society of America Tenth Annual Meeting*, 1979.

16. Mullinix JM, Norton BJ, Hack S, Fishman MA: Skin temperature biofeedback and migraine. *Headache* 17:242–244, 1978.

17. Hadfield TA: The influence of suggestion on body temperature. *Lancet* 2:68–69, 1920.

18. Taub E, Emurian CS: Operant control of skin temperature. Presented to Biofeedback Research Society Annual Meeting, 1971.

19. Asterita MF, Fedorchak FN: Variation in peripheral body temperature during self-regulation of dominant hand temperature. *Proceedings of Biofeedback Society of America Annual Meeting*, 1979.

20. Kaplan BJ, Crawford DG: Target training: a technique for assessing self-regulation of skin temperature. *Biofeedback and Self-Regulation* 4(1), 1979.

21. Taub E, Emurian CS: Feedback-aided self-regulation of skin temperature with a single feedback locus: 1. Acquisition and reversal training. *Biofeedback and Self-Regulation* 1(2):147–168, 1976.

22. Thompson D: Learning voluntary control of fingertip skin temperature: Issues, questions, and answers. *Proceedings of Biofeedback Research Society Annual Meeting*, 1976.

23. Werbach MR, Sandweiss JH: Peripheral temperatures of migraineurs undergoing relaxation training. *Headache* 18(4):211–217, 1978.

24. Roberts AH, Kewman DG, MacDonald H: Voluntary control of skin temperature: Unilateral changes using hypnosis and feedback. *J Abnorm Psychol* 82(1):163–168, 1973.
25. Roberts AH, Schuler J, Bacon JR, Zimmerman RL, Patterson P: Individual differences and autonomic control: Absorption, hypnotic susceptibility and the unilateral control of skin temperature. *J Abnorm Psychol* 84:272–279, 1975.
26. Maslach C, Marshall G, Zimbardo PG: Hypnotic control of peripheral skin temperature: A case report. *Psychophysiology* 9:600–605, 1972.
27. Turin AC: Biofeedback and suggestion in finger temperature training: An effect for the controls but not the "treatments." *Biofeedback and Self-Regulation* 2:296, 1977.
28. Keefe FJ: Conditioning changes in differential skin temperature. *Percept Mot Skills* 40:283–288, 1975.
29. Leeb C, French D, Fahrion S: The effect of instructional set on autogenic biofeedback hand temperature training. *Proceedings of Biofeedback Research Society Annual Meeting*, 1974.
30. Thompson C: Autogenic feedback training: The effects of outcome and accessibility of hand temperature biofeedback on the reduction of migraine headaches. *Diss Abstr Int* 37(7-B), 3635B–3636B, 1977.
31. Mathew RJ, Claghorn JL, Meyer JS, Largen J, Dobbins K: Relationship between volitional alteration in skin temperature and regional cerebral blood flow in normal subjects. *Proceedings of Biofeedback Society of America Ninth Annual Meeting*, 1978.
32. Largen JW, Mathew RJ, Dobbins K, Meyer JS, Sakai F, Claghorn JL: The effect of direction of skin temperature self-regulation on migraine activity and regional cerebral blood flow. *Proceedings of Biofeedback Society of America Tenth Annual Meeting*, 1979.
33. Sovak M, Kunzel M, Sternbach RA, Dalessio DJ: Is volitional manipulation of hemodynamics a valid rationale for biofeedback therapy of migraine? *Headache* 18:197–202, 1978.
34. Koppman JW, McDonald RD, Kunzel MG: Voluntary regulation of a temporal artery diameter by migraine patients. *Headache* 14:133–138, 1974.
35. Savill GE, Koppman JW: Voluntary temporal artery regulation compared with finger blood volume and temperature. *Proceedings of Biofeedback Research Society Sixth Annual Meeting*, 1975.
36. Friar LR, Beatty J: Migraine: Management by trained control of vasoconstriction *Consult Clin Psychol* 44(1):46–53, 1976.
37. Zamani R: Treatment of migraine headache: Biofeedback versus deep muscle relaxation. *Research Report*, PR 785–2. Minneapolis, University of Minnesota Medical School, 1975.
38. Bild R: Cephalic vasomotor response biofeedback as a treatment modality for vascular headache of the migraine type. *Diss Abstr Int* 37(5-B), 2494B (abstract), 1976.
39. Feuerstein M, Adams H: Cephalic vasomotor feedback in the modification of migraine headaches. *Biofeedback and Self-Regulation* 2(3):241–254, 1977.

40. Price KP, Tursky B: Vascular reactivity of migraineurs and non-migraineurs: A comparison of responses to self-control procedures. *Headache* 16:210–217, 1976.
41. Bakal DA, Kaganov JA: Muscle-contraction and migraine headache: Psychophysiological comparison. *Headache* 17:208–215, 1977.
42. Mitchell KR: The treatment of migraine: An exploratory application of time-limited behavior therapy. *Technology* 14:50, 1969.
43. Mitchell KR, Mitchell DM: Migraine: Exploratory treatment application of programmed behavior therapy techniques. *J Psychosom Res* 15:137–159, 1971.
44. Hay KM, Madders J: Migraine treated by relaxation therapy. *J R Coll Gen Pract* 21:664, 1971.
45. Blanchard EB, Theobald DE, Brown DA, Silver BV, Williamson DA: A controlled comparison of temperature biofeedback and autogenic training with progressive relaxation training in the treatment of migraine headaches. Presented to Biofeedback Society of America Annual Meeting, 1977.
46. Silver BV, Blanchard EB, Williamson DA, Theobald DE, Brown DA: Temperature biofeedback and relaxation training in the treatment of migraine headaches. One year follow-up. *Biofeedback and Self-Regulation* 4(4), 1979.
47. Luthe W, Schultz JH: *Autogenic Therapy*, vol 2: *Medical Applications*. New York, Grune & Stratton, 1969.
48. Fahrion SL: Autogenic biofeedback treatment for migraine. *Mayo Clin Proc* 52:776–784, 1977.
49. Baudewyns PA: A comparison of the effects of stress versus relaxation instruction on the finger temperature response. *Behavior Therapy* 7:54–67, 1976.
50. Scott J. Timmons B: On the relationship between frontalis EMG activity and skin temperature: A preliminary model with very little data. *Proceedings of Biofeedback Research Society Annual Meeting*, 1974.
51. Diamond S, Franklin M: Indications and contraindications for the use of biofeedback therapy in headache patients. *Proceedings of Biofeedback Research Society Annual Meeting*, 1974.
52. Medina JL, Diamond S, Franklin M: Biofeedback therapy for migraine. *Headache* 16(3):418, 1976.
53. Diamond S, Franklin M: Biofeedback—choice of treatment in childhood migraine, in Luthe W, Antonelli F (eds): *Therapy in Psychosomatic Medicine*, vol 4, *Autogenic Therapy*. Rome, 1977.
54. Diamond S, Diamond-Falk J, DeVeno T: The value of biofeedback in the treatment of chronic headache: A five-year retrospective study. *Proceedings of Biofeedback Research Society Annual Meeting*, 1978.
55. Fried FE, Lamberti J, Sneed P: Treatment of tension and migraine headaches with biofeedback techniques. *Mo Med* 74(6):253–255, 1977.
56. Hartje JC, Diver CE: Variation in hand temperature as a correlate to migraine severity. *Proceedings of Biofeedback Society of America Ninth Annual Meeting*, 1978.
57. Pozniak-Patewicz E: Cephalgic spasm of head and neck muscles. Sandoz-Information, *Proceedings of Bergen Migraine Symposium*, suppl. 1, 61, 1975.

58. Beasley J: Biofeedback in the treatment of migraine headaches. *Diss Abstr Int* 36 (11-B), 5850B–5851B (abstract), 1976.
59. Adler CS, Adler SM: The pragmatic application of biofeedback to headaches: A 5-year clinical follow-up. Presented to Biofeedback Research Society Annual Meeting, 1976.
60. Boller JD, Flom RP: Treatment of the common migraine: Systematic application of biofeedback and autogenic training. *Proceedings of Biofeedback Society of America Annual Meeting*, 1978.
61. Werbach MR, Sandweiss JH: Finger temperature characteristics of migraineurs undergoing biofeedback assisted relaxation training. *Proceedings of Biofeedback Society of America Ninth Annual Meeting*, 1978.
62. Weinstock SA: A tentative procedure for the control of pain: Migraine and tension headaches. *Proceedings of Biofeedback Research Society Annual Meeting*, 1972.
63. Gannon L, Sternbach RA: Alpha enhancement as treatment for pain: A case study. *Journal of Behavior Therapy and Experimental Psychiatry* 2:209–213, 1971.
64. Melzack R, Perry C: Self-regulation of pain: The use of alpha-feedback and hypnotic training for the control of chronic pain, in Wickramasekera I (ed): *Biofeedback Behavior Therapy and Hypnosis: Potentiating the Verbal Control of Behavior for Clinicians.* Chicago, Nelson-Hall, 1976.
65. Kasanof D: Biofeedback therapy with electronic teaching aids. *Patient Care* August 1, 1975.
66. Andreychuk T, Skriver C: Hypnosis and biofeedback in the treatment of migraine headache. Presented to Biofeedback Research Society Annual Meeting, 1974.
67. Cohen MJ, Levee JR, McArthur DL, Rickles WH: Physiological and psychological dimensions of migraine headache and biofeedback training. *Biofeedback and Self-Regulation* 1(3), 1976.
68. Graham G: Hypnosis and biofeedback as treatments for migraine headaches. *Diss Abstr Int* 35 (5-B), 2428B–2429B (abstract), 1974.
69. Crosson B, Andreychuk T, Tiemann K, Phillips C: Combined use of hypnosis and biofeedback in the treatment of migraines: A pilot study. *Biofeedback and Self-Regulation* 3(2):240, 1978.
70. Taub E: Self-regulation of human tissue temperature, in Schwartz GE, Beatty J (eds): *Biofeedback: Theory and Research.* New York, Academic Press, in press, chapter 11.
71. Price KP: The application of behavior therapy to the treatment of psychosomatic disorders: Retrospect and prospect. *Psychotherapy: Theory, Research, and Practice* 2(2), 1974.
72. Blanchard EB, Young LD: Clinical applications of biofeedback training. *Arch Gen Psychiatry* 30:573–589, 1974.
73. Jessup BA, Neufeld RWJ, Merskey H: Biofeedback therapy for headache and other pain: An evaluative review. *Pain* 7:225–270, 1979.
74. Miller NE: Biofeedback and visceral learning. *Ann Rev Psychol* 29:373–404, 1978.

75. Barber TX: Introduction. Self-control; temperature biofeedback, in *Biofeedback and Self-control*. Chicago, Aldine, 1975.
76. Stroebel CF, Glueck BC: Psychophysiological rationale for the application of biofeedback in the alleviation of pain, in *Pain*. New York, Plenum, 1976.
77. Kentsmith D, Strider F, Copenhauer J, Jacques D: Effects of biofeedback upon the suppression of migraine symptoms and plasma dopamine-beta-hydroxylase activity. *Headache* 16:173–177, 1976.
78. Gaardner KR, Montgomery P: Clinical biofeedback: A procedure manual. Baltimore, Williams & Wilkins, 1977, p 51.
79. Birk L (ed): *Biofeedback: Behavioral Medicine*. New York, Grune & Stratton, 1973, pp 51–53.
80. Wickramasekera I: *Biofeedback, Behavior Therapy, and Hypnosis: Potentiating the Verbal Control of Behavior for Clinicians*. Chicago, Nelson-Hall, 1976.
81. Diamond S, Baltes BJ: The diagnosis and treatment of headaches. *Chicago Medical School Quarterly* 32:1–4, 1973.
82. Diamond S, Franklin M: Autogenic training and biofeedback in treatment of chronic headache problems in adults, in Luthe W, Antonelli F (eds): *Therapy in Psychosomatic Medicine. Proceedings of Third Congress of International College of Psychosomatic Medicine*, Rome, 1975.
83. Fordyce WE, Fowler RS, Lehmann JF, DeLateur BJ: Operant conditioning in the treatment of chronic pain. *Arch Phys Med Rehabil* 54:399–408, 1973.
84. Budzynski T: Biofeedback procedures in the clinic, in Birk L (ed): *Biofeedback: Behavioral Medicine*. New York, Grune & Stratton, 1973.
85. Diamond S, Franklin M: Autogenic training with biofeedback in children with migraine, in Luthe W, Antonelli F (eds): *Therapy in Psychosomatic Medicine. Proceedings of Third Congress of International College of Psychosomatic Medicine*, Rome, 1975.
86. Feuerstein M, Adams HE, Beiman I: Cephalic vasomotor and electromyographic feedback in the treatment of combined muscle-contraction and migraine headaches in a geriatric case. *Headache* 16:232–237, 1976.
87. Diamond S, Franklin M: Intensive biofeedback therapy in the treatment of headache. *Proceedings of Biofeedback Research Society Sixth Annual Meeting*, 1975.

Copyright © 1981, Spectrum Publications, Inc.
Treatment of Migraine

Chapter 5
Biochemistry of Migraine

LEE KUDROW, M.D.

Migraine is considered a vasomotor disorder. Even during periods between headaches, migraineurs have demonstrated increased reactivity of blood vessels. Frequently patients complain of the persistent coldness of their hands and feet, especially during minimally stressful periods. This tendency of peripheral vasoconstriction has been documented [1]. More profound vascular changes have been recorded during the prodromal and painful stages of classical migraine. O'Brien [2] and others [3–6] reported that specific cerebral blood flow (CBF) changes occurred during these stages; CBF was found to be decreased during the prodrome and increased during pain. Skinhøj and Paulson [3] suggested that transient cerebral ischemia was associated with the prodromal phase of migraine and approached that of carotid occlusive disease. Indeed, Welch et al. [7] had demonstrated altered levels of gamma-aminobutyric acid (GABA) and cyclic AMP in spinal fluid of migraineurs, associating these changes with the effects of ischemia.

Although vascular changes in migraine are of considerable interest, they are not the primary cause of the development of migraine. One should look at the biochemical events found to be associated with this disorder.

In recent years, several biochemical pathways of migraine have been identified. It is not certain whether these biochemical changes are primary or secondary to the disorder. Nevertheless, models constructed from these findings help to explain the relationship of environmental influences to the vasomotor changes seen in migraine. These models have helped to identify specific pain mechanisms.

BIOCHEMICAL MECHANISMS

Serotonin

The importance of biogenic amines in migraine, specifically serotonin (5-HT), was introduced by Sicuteri et al. [8] in 1961. They found that during migraine attacks hydroxyindoleacetic acid excretion was increased. This finding stimulated a renewed interest in migraine as a vasomotor disorder, emphasizing biochemical rather than neurogenic mechanisms.

In 1967, Anthony et al. [9] published their landmark paper on plasma serotonin changes in classical migraine. They found that blood platelet serotonin levels were significantly increased during the prodromal stage and decreased during the headache phase of migraine. These results confirmed those of Sicuteri et al. [8] and provided information on the more proximal serotonin changes associated with the migraine attack. Specifically, Lance et al. [10] showed that serotonin had a strong constrictor effect on extracranial arteries and, experimentally, it was capable of aborting the migraine attack.

The role of serotonin in migraine was further elucidated by platelet studies of Kalendovsky and Austin [11] and subsequently confirmed by Deshmukh and Meyer [12]. The latter authors found that during the headache-free state, migraineurs showed a significantly lower circulating microemboli index and higher aggregation. Platelet adhesiveness and aggregation increased during the prodrome, whereas, during the headache phase, adhesiveness increased significantly, while aggregation decreased [12]. These findings correlated with plasma serotonin changes for both phases of migraine, as had been demonstrated earlier [9].

Free Fatty Acids

Other biochemical changes were found to participate in the development of migraine. In 1970, Hockaday et al. [13] reported that during migraine attacks, free fatty acids (FFA) plasma levels were increased. Corroborating these findings, Anthony [14] subsequently reported that FFA levels increased by 10 to 174 percent among migraineurs during attacks and were significantly higher than during preheadache and postheadache phases. Stress resulting from pain was ruled out as the stimulus for plasma FFA elevation, since no significant mean rise occurred in two controlled populations subjected to similar stresses (cluster attacks and pneumoencephalographic procedures). The importance of FFA changes is apparent in light of the role of prostaglandins in migraine.

Prostaglandins (PG)

Prostaglandins are of considerable interest in migraine, in that they are vasomotor substances and also play a major role in platelet activity. In other words, prostaglandins affect blood vessel changes directly and indirectly. As has been pointed out by Horrobin [15], PGE1, when injected into nonmigraine subjects, caused migraine-like headaches [16]. As a potent extracranial vasodilator, PGE1 may cause an internal carotid artery steal, as Welch and his associates [17] demonstrated in their innovative carotid artery blood-flow studies in monkeys. Substances known to influence migraine attacks, such as serotonin, phenylethylamine, and tyramine, stimulate PG release from the lungs. Further, this release is inhibited by the ergotamines. Sandler [18] considered this prostaglandin release phenomenon an important step in migraine pathogenesis.

The precursors of prostaglandin synthesis are the free fatty acids. Prostaglandin endoperoxide is synthesized from arachidonic acid and in the platelets produces thromboxane A2 via platelet enzyme activity. Thromboxane A2 reduces cyclic AMP levels, resulting in a shape change of the platelets. This leads to the release of serotonin, thromboxane, beta-thromboglobulin (BTG), and other substances. This release reaction is ultimately responsible for platelet aggregation [19].

In the vessel wall, prostacycline is synthesized from the enzymatic action of cyclo-oxygenase on prostaglandin endoperoxide. Prostacycline increases platelet cyclic AMP following contact of the platelet and vessel wall. This inhibits shape change and the subsequent aggregation of platelets (Figure 1). Thus, homeostasis of platelet activity seems to be depen-

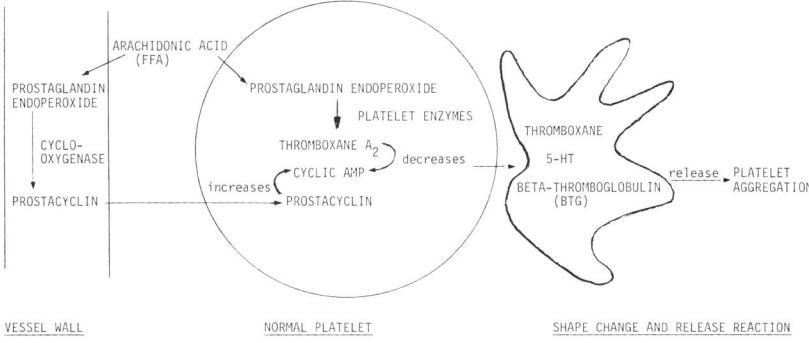

Figure 1. Major biochemical pathways of platelet aggregation.

dent, at least in part, on the balance of prostacycline and thromboxane activity, both products of prostaglandin [20]. Recently Gawel et al. [21] demonstrated significantly increased plasma levels of BTG during migraine attacks, a finding consistent with the aforementioned biochemical and platelet changes.

Monoamine Oxidase

Another biochemical marker of migraine is monoamine oxidase (MAO), MAOB in particular. This is of special interest, since MAOB is a platelet constituent. In 1970, Sandler and his colleagues [22] found an MAOB deficiency in some migraineurs. This study was prompted by the findings of Hanington [23] who had documented tyramine induction in some patients. This suggested enzyme (monoamine oxidase) deficiency. Subsequently phenylethylamine-oxidizing deficiency was also incriminated in dietary migraine [24]. Sicuteri et al. [25] reported platelet MAO deficit in migraine, confirming the earlier findings of Sandler et al. [22].

A scheme incorporating these biochemical changes as they influence platelet aggregation, and ultimately serotonin release, is presented in Figure 2. Increased FFAs, resulting from fasting, stress, or amine loads, increase prostaglandin synthesis. Plasma amine concentrations are increased in the presence of MAOB deficiency. Estrogens may stimulate the secretion of prostaglandins directly or through prolactin secretion, as will be discussed later. Finally, platelet aggregation occurs through the prostaglandin endoperoxide-thromboxane A2 pathway (Figure 2).

Estrogens

Estrogen is clearly a major influence in migraine. Effects of extrinsic estrogen on migraine frequency have been clinically observed and documented [26–28]. In a study of 239 women with migraine, of whom 60 used oral contraceptives, 87 were treated with cyclic supplemental estrogens, and 92 did not use hormones, a significantly increased headache frequency was noted in the estrogen-using groups. Moreover, when the women stopped taking pills, their headache frequency decreased by 80 percent. Similarly, reduction and "decycling" of estrogen supplements resulted in a 70 percent improvement [28].

In a small population of women with menstrual migraine (headaches associated with menses or premenses), Sommerville [29] demonstrated a relationship between menstrual migraine attacks and changing estrogen levels.

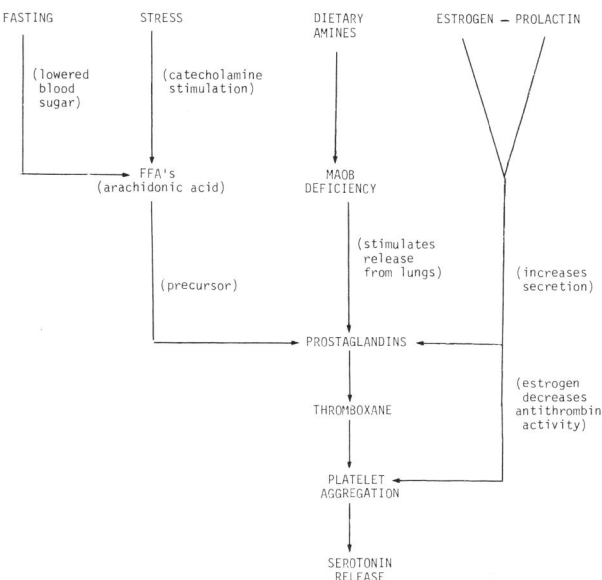

Figure 2. Migraine pathogenesis (part 1): The influence of environmental factors on the prostaglandin-serotonin pathway.

Prevalence of migraine is greater in females than in males. That intrinsic estrogen changes are responsible for this is further suggested by comparison of female to male ratios of migraine in pre- and postpubescent ages. In childhood this ratio is 1:1 [30], whereas in adults it is 3:1 [31].

Estrogen exerts its influence on migraine through its effects on platelet function. Estrogens increase plasma antiplasmin activity, decrease serum antithrombin activity [32], increase platelet aggregation [33], and stimulate prostaglandin secretion directly [34] and indirectly, by stimulating prolactin secretion [35] (Figure 3).

Basophil Cell Heparin

From a series of studies Thonnard-Neumann [36–39] concluded that migraine is associated with a deficiency in native heparin. Migraineurs, he found, have fewer basophilic leukocytes and the cells contained less heparin than did those of controls. Furthermore, these changes were associated with high plasma levels of low-density lipoproteins and reduced

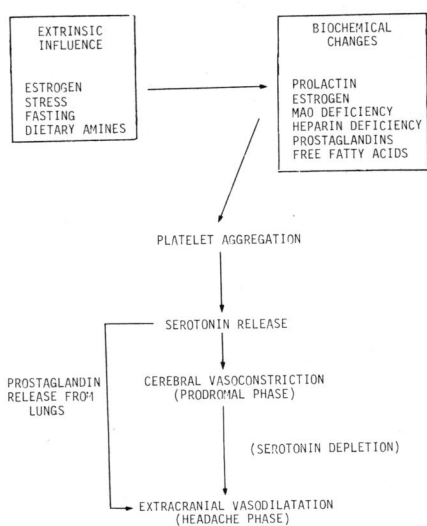

Figure 3. Migraine pathogenesis (part 2): Serotonin influences on vascular changes.

excretion of uroheparin. Periodic administration of heparin by either intravenous injection or aerosol inhalation reversed these changes and reduced the frequency and severity of migraine attacks. He stated that heparin stabilizes migraine by reducing platelet adhesiveness, directly or indirectly interfering with vasoactive amines, and by clearing plasma lipids.

PAIN MECHANISMS

There are currently two concepts of the pain mechanisms of migraine. The first holds that the site of migraine pain is in the periphery. In this scheme the initial pathways involve many of the biochemical changes discussed earlier. Thus serotonin released from aggregated platelets is responsible for the cerebral vasoconstriction of the prodromal phase of migraine. Serotonin activates the release of prostaglandin from the lungs, and the subsequent serotonin depletion causes painful extracranial vasodilatation (the headache phase). Central serotonin depletion may also lead to a reduced pain threshold.

BIOCHEMISTRY OF MIGRAINE

Fanchamps [40] includes a second pathway system which is activated concurrent to platelet release of serotonin. He suggests that mast cells liberate histamine and proteolytic enzymes. The combined effect of histamine and serotonin increases capillary permeability. This facilitates transudation of plasmakinins, formed by the action of proteolytic enzymes on plasmakininogen, into blood vessel walls and perivascular tissue.

The net result of these reactions is peripherally painful vasodilatation and increased sensitivity of vessel walls and perivascular tissue, all enhanced by a lowered pain threshold (Figure 4).

The second and most recent theory concerned with migraine pain mechanisms is that of Sicuteri and his coworkers [41, 42]. Sicuteri [43] rejected the proposal that migraine pain was mediated by peripheral vasodilatation. Nor did he find it creditable that pain-producing substances, such as kinins, serotonin, prostaglandin, etc. were concentrated sufficiently at the peripheral sites to account for the pain of migraine. He believed rather that migraine represented a disorder characterized by a lower pain threshold, due to a failure of central modulation-inhibition of pain, that is, deficient nociception.

Sicuteri [43] further hypothesized that the central monoamine turnover deficiency could cause increased sensitivity of the receptor on which the specific mediator acts. In a series of experiments with migraine patients, in which venous spasm of the dorsal hand vein was measured in response to injection of specific monoamines, Sicuteri and co-workers [44] demonstrated the expected supersensitivity responses. These were

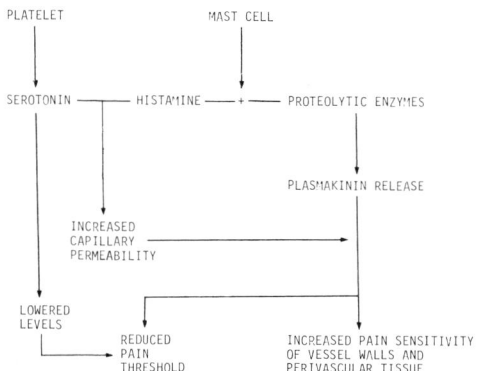

Figure 4. Migraine pathogenesis (part 3): Pain mechanisms influenced by mast cell and platelet changes.

found for receptors of 5-HT, dopamine, noradrenaline, and tyramine. Fanciullaci [45] also demonstrated an adrenergic impairment in the iris of migraineurs.

CONCLUSION

We may conclude that, because of inherent enzyme deficiencies, much as yet unknown, abnormal biochemical reactivity occurs in response to extrinsic and intrinsic environmental changes. Thus, migraine appears to be a disorder characterized by deficiencies of adaptation mechanisms.

It is clear that migraine is a multisystemic disorder involving peripheral and central mechanisms. From investigative and clinical standpoints, multidisciplinary interest is required to achieve satisfactory understanding and treatment of the disorder.

REFERENCES

1. Price KP, Tursky B: Vascular reactivity of migraineurs and nonmigraineurs: A comparison of responses to self-control procedures. *Headache* 16:210–217, 1976.
2. O'Brien MD: Cerebral cortex perfusion rates in migraine. *Lancet* 1:1036, 1967.
3. Skinhøj E, Paulson OB: Regional blood flow in internal carotid distribution during migraine attack. *Br Med J* 3:569–570, 1969.
4. Norris JW, Hachinski VC, Cooper PW: Changes in cerebral blood flow during a migraine attack. *Br Med J* 3:676–677, 1975.
5. Mathew NT, Hrastnik F, Meyer JS: Regional cerebral blood flow in the diagnosis of vascular headache. *Headache* 15:252–260, 1976.
6. Sakai F, Meyer JS: Regional cerebral hemodynamics during migraine and cluster headaches measured by the ^{133}Xe inhalation method. *Headache* 18:122–132, 1978.
7. Welch KMA, Chabi E, Nell JH, Bartosh K, Chee ANA, Mathew NT, Achar VS: Biochemical comparison of migraine and stroke. *Headache* 16:160–167, 1976.
8. Sicuteri F, Testi A, Anselmi B: Biochemical investigations in headache: Increase in the hydroxyindoleacetic acid excretion during migraine attacks. *Int Arch Allergy Appl Immunol* 19:55–58, 1961.
9. Anthony M, Hinterberger H, Lance JW: Plasma serotonin in migraine and stress. *Arch Neurol* 16:544–552, 1967.
10. Lance JW, Anthony M, and Gorski A: Serotonin, the carotid body, and cranial vessels in migraine. *Arch Neurol* 16:553, 1967.
11. Kalendovsky, Z, Austin JH: "Complicated migraine," its association with increased platelet aggregability and abnormal plasma coagulation factors. *Headache* 15:18–35, 1975.

12. Deshmukh SV, Meyer JS: Cyclic changes in platelet dynamics and the pathogenesis and prophylaxis of migraine. *Headache* 17:101–108, 1977.
13. Hockaday JM, Williamson DH, Whitty CWM: Blood glucose levels and fatty acid metabolism in migraine related to fasting. *Lancet* 2:1153–1156, 1970.
14. Anthony M: Plasma free fatty acids and prostaglandin E, in migraine and stress. *Headache* 16:58–63, 1976.
15. Horrobin DF: Prostaglandins and migraine. *Headache* 17:113–117, 1977.
16. Carlsen LA, Ekelund LG, Oro L: Chemical and metabolic effects of prostaglandin E1 in man. *Acta Med Scand* 183:423–430, 1968.
17. Welch KMA, Spira PJ, Knowles L, Lance JW: Effects of prostaglandins on the internal and external carotid blood flow in the monkey. *Neurology* 24:705–710, 1974.
18. Sandler M: Migraine: A pulmonary disease? *Lancet* 1:618–619, 1972.
19. Hanberg M, Svensson J, and Samuelsson B: Thromboxanes, a new group of biologically active compounds derived from prostaglandin endoperoxides. *Proc Natl Acad Sci USA* 72:2994–2998, 1975.
20. Moncada S, Vane JR: Unstable metabolites of arachidonic acid and their role in haemostasis and thrombosis. *Br Med Bull* 34:129–135, 1978.
21. Gawel M, Burkitt M, Rose FC: The platelet release reaction during migraine attacks. *Headache* 19:323–327, 1979.
22. Sandler M, Youdim MBH, Southgate J, Hanington E: The role of tyramine in migraine: Some possible biochemical mechanisms, in Cochrane AL (ed): *Background to Migraine*, Third Migraine Symposium, London, Heinemann, 1970, p 103.
23. Hanington E: Preliminary report on tyramine headache. *Br Med J* 2:550–551, 1967.
24. Sandler M, Youdim MBH, Hanington E: A phenylethylamine-oxydising defect in migraine. *Nature* 250:335–337, 1974.
25. Sicuteri F, Buffoni F, Anselmi B, Del Bianco PL: An enzyme (MAO) defect in platelets in migraine. *Res Clin Stud Headache* 3:245–251, 1972.
26. Grant ECG: Relation between headaches from oral contraceptives and development of endometrial arterioles. *Br Med J* 3:402–405, 1968.
27. Whitty CWM, Hockaday JM, Whitty MM: The effect of oral contraceptives on migraine. *Lancet* 1:856–859, 1966.
28. Kudrow L: The relationship of headache frequency to hormone use in migraine. *Headache* 15:35–40, 1975.
29. Sommerville BW: The role of estradiol withdrawal in the etiology of menstrual migraine. *Neurology* 22:355–365, 1972.
30. Krupp GR, Friedman AP: Migraine in children: A report of fifty children. Presented to American Medical Association, Chicago, June 1950.
31. Waters WE, O'Connor PJ: Prevalence of migraine. *J Neurol Neurosurg Psychiatry* 30:613–616, 1975.
32. Howie PW, Mallinson AC, Prentice CRM, et al: Effect of combined oestrogen-progesterone oral contraceptive, oestrogen, and progesterone on antiplasmin and antithrombin activity. *Lancet* 2:1329–1332, 1970.

33. Mettler L, Selchow BM: Oral contraceptives and platelet function. *Thrombos Diathes Haemorrh* 29:213–220, 1972.
34. Castracane VD, Jordan VC: Considerations into the mechanism of estrogen-stimulated prostaglandin synthesis. *Prostaglandins* 12:243–251, 1976.
35. Horrobin DF: *Prolactin: Physiology and Chemical Significance.* Lancaster, Medical and Technical Publishing Company, 1973.
36. Thonnard-Neumann E, Taylor WL: The basophilic leukocyte and migraine. *Headache* 8:98–107, 1968.
37. Thonnard-Neumann E: Some interrelationships of vasoactive substances and basophilic leukocytes in migraine headaches. *Headache* 9:130–140, 1969.
38. Thonnard-Neumann E: Heparin in migraine headache. *Headache* 13:49–64, 1973.
39. Thonnard-Neumann E: Migraine therapy with heparin: Pathophysiologic basis. *Headache* 16:284–292, 1977.
40. Fanchamps A: The role of humoral mediators in migraine headache. *Can J Neurol Sci* 1:189–195, 1974.
41. Sicuteri F: Headache as a possible expression of deficiency of brain 5-hydroxy-tryptamine (central denervation supersensitivity). *Headache* 12:69–72, 1972.
42. Sicuteri F, Anselmi B, Del Bianco PL: 5-Hydroxytryptamine supersensitivity as a new theory of headache and central pain: A clinical pharmacological approach with *p*-chlorophenylalanine. *Psychopharmacologia (Berlin)* 29:347, 1973.
43. Sicuteri F: Headache as a metonymy of non-organic central pain, in Sicuteri F (ed): *Headache New Vistas.* Florence, Italy, Biomedical Press, 1977, pp 19–67.
44. Sicuteri F, Anselmi B, Del Bianco PL: Systemic non-organic central pain: A new syndrome with decentralization supersensitivity. *Headache* 18:133–136, 1978.
45. Fanciullaci M: Iris adrenergic impairment in idiopathic headache. *Headache* 19:8–13, 1979.

Chapter 6

Integration of Psychosomatic Self-Regulation of Headache into Medically Recognized Therapies

JOSEPH D. SARGENT, M.D.

The important mileposts in medicine have often occurred unannounced and seemingly by accident. They usually have been preceded, however, by a series of experiences that made an investigator alert to the meaning of a serendipitous event. The discovery of penicillin by Fleming, which ushered in the era of antibiotic therapy, is an example. Such events ultimately lead to a feverish pace of research activity. Gradually a wealth of contradictory experience emerges, fueled by different perspectives, but ultimately a consensus develops. At this time the application of thermal training to migraine remains in the investigational phase without agreement on its worth. Such a consensus will not develop for nondrug therapies for headache until they are confirmed by biochemical and physiological observations. However, the absence of a clear understanding of an etiological mechanism for migraine makes its difficult to develop a consensus. My main purposes are to develop a theory of how psychosomatic self-regulation of the hand vasculature might help migraine patients and to show how this treatment modality may be integrated with medically recognized therapies for migraine.

HISTORICAL PERSPECTIVE

Graham and Wolff [1] were the first to show that pulsation of the temporal artery is increased during the headache phase. Their work was based on observations of the effects of ergotamine tartrate on extracranial vessels in relieving migraine attacks. Ergotamine tartrate diminished the increased amplitude of the arterial pulse with corresponding relief of the headache. These results seemed reasonable in view of previous work with histamine, which had clearly shown that stretched extracranial arteries are capable of producing pain [2, 3].

Schumacher and Wolff [4], working on methods to increase intracranial pressure and the administration of amyl nitrite, observed: "The essential migraine phenomena result from dysfunction of cranial arteries and represent contrasts in vascular mechanisms and vascular beds. Preheadache disturbances follow occlusive vasoconstriction of cerebral arteries, while the headache results from dilation and distension chiefly of branches of external carotid arteries."

A chance cerebral angiogram done on a patient by Dukes and Vieth [5] during a classical migraine attack showed a diminution in the caliber of the internal carotid system with reflux into the vertebral vessels during the prodromal phase. At the beginning of the headache phase, blood flow returned to normal.

Through measurements of regional cerebral blood flow (rCBF) by the inhalation of ^{133}Xenon, Edmeads [6] showed that there is decreased bilateral rCBF during the migraine aura which is usually most marked in that portion of the brain corresponding to the aura. This reduction in certain areas may last into the headache phase while other portions of the brain are hyperperfused. Such areas have shown up as edema and infarction on computed axial tomography (CAT) scans. The hyperperfusion of the intracranial vasculature may outlast the headache by more than two days; however, the hyperperfusion in the extracranial vasculature subsides promptly when the headache disappears.

Wolff [7] proposed that vasodilation of the cerebral circulation occurs whenever an adequate blood supply to the brain is endangered. If cerebrovascular dilation is great enough, the extracranial arteries will dilate and release chemical factors, producing edema and lowering pain threshold. What initiates vasoconstriction is not clear.

In recent years investigators have postulated that an agent (or agents) causing vasoconstriction may be released to start the headache sequence. Sicuteri [8] proposed that the liberated chemical substances are amines, such as norepinephrine, epinephrine, or serotonin, all powerful vasoconstrictors. Other biochemical agents implicated in the headache sequence are acetylcholine, adenosine, triphosphate, bradykinin, and histamine. In the migraine attack, some subjects have excreted increased amounts of catecholamine end products, particularly 5-hydroxyindole acetic acid from serotonin and 4-hydroxy-3-methoxy-D-mandelic acid (VMA) from nonrepinephrine and epinephrine. Lance et al. [9] have shown a corresponding reduction in blood serotonin levels.

Because the migraine syndrome is a multifaceted disorder, some investigators have postulated a dysfunction in the hypothalamus as the provocative element in the attack. Thus, Pearce [10] suggested that the hypothalamus may profoundly influence the autonomic control of the peripheral vasculature. Pearce postulated a periodic central disturbance of hypothalamic activity or labile threshold which accounts for the periodicity of the migraine attack and provides a mechanism for emotional disturbances to be mediated by pathways from the limbic system to the hypothalamus.

From three groups of clinical manifestations, Herberg [11] proposed an etiological role in migraine headaches determined by the variation of hypothalamic activity. The groups are: peripheral vasomotor involvement, as seen in the temporal arteries, conjunctiva, and skin; metabolic and vegetative disturbance, such as variations in water balance, food intake, mood, and sleep; and "accentuated secondary drives" of the migraine personality, which have been related to hypothalamic activity. Rao and Pearce [12] failed to demonstrate a disturbance in the hypothalamic-pituitary-adrenal axis of migraine subjects, using metyrapone and insulin hypoglycemia tests. However, a consistently observed pattern of "hypoglycemia-unresponsiveness" suggested a possible hypothalamic dysfunction.

In a later article Herberg [13] stated, "there seems little doubt that migraine is ultimately a circulatory disturbance in which spasms of the cerebral blood vessels, succeeded by dilatation, are associated with an excessive and painful dilatation of separate vessels in the adjacent scalp." Regarding the sympathetic nerve supply originating in the spinal cord, he pointed out that "close examination has shown that the sympathetic supply comes to an abrupt end soon after small arteries have penetrated the substance of the brain. It has been assumed, therefore, that the sympathetic nerve supply can play little or no direct role in the normal regulation of cerebral blood flow or in disorders of the cerebral circulation such as migraine." The main supply of norepinephrine in the brain emanates from neural pathways that originate in the locus coeruleus, which is the largest norepinephrine-producing nucleus within the mammalian brain. However, the main supply of norepinephrine fibers to the hypothalamus comes from brainstem norepinephrine cell groups, called the lateral tegmental norepinephrine system. In fact, the principal target of this system is the medial portion of the hypothalamus which has a significant role in the regulation of gonadotropin, growth hormone, and ACTH secretion. What activates this system is unknown, but it is clear that the cerebral vasculature does have a sympathetic nerve supply.

One could extend Herberg's hypothesis, that overactivity of the hypothalamus is the primary site of disturbance in the migraine syndrome, involving overactivity of the entire catecholamine system of the central nervous system. Biochemical evidence is provided by a previous statement made by Sicuteri [8] regarding metabolites of catecholamine and serotonin which are found in increased amounts in urine during the headache phase. There is a plausible explanation, therefore, for the lack of totally preventive medications: present medications used for prevention of a migraine attack only inhibit one portion of the total system. Examples are methysergide, a serotonin antagonist, and propranolol, a beta-adrenergic blocker. Actually, the most effective treatment would be one that would have an effect on all catecholamine systems, and such a treatment might be psychosomatic self-regulation.

Kentsmith et al. [14] demonstrated a simultaneous reduction in one subject's symptoms and plasma dopamine-beta-hyroxylase activity through concentrative, meditation, thermal, and relaxation training. The decrease in dopamine-beta-hydroxylase supposedly reflects suppression of autonomic activity. Perhaps activation of the cerebral cortex can inhibit the activity of the catecholamine system.

Mathew et al. [15] have shown a decrease in platelet monoamine oxidase activity during relaxation therapy, which provides additional support to the speculation that cortical activation may inhibit the sympathetic nervous system.

RATIONALE FOR PSYCHOSOMATIC SELF-REGULATION

Miller [16] presented research that challenges the concept that "learning" in the autonomic nervous system is a reflection of skeletal muscle activity. He showed that heart rate, gastrointestinal contractions, blood pressure, and the rate of saliva and urine formation in animals can be directly controlled through operant conditioning techniques via the autonomic nervous system. In human beings, there is scientific evidence of voluntary control of the autonomic nervous system through autogenic training as well as in the training techniques of Yoga [17, 18].

Autogenic training, according to Schultz and Luthe [18], is a therapeutic method that involves the simultaneous regulation of mental and somatic functions. The desired somatic responses are brought about by conscious thought using preselected phrases. The specific responses brought under voluntary control during preliminary training are heaviness in the limbs, warmth in the extremities, control of heart rate, sense of warmth in the abdomen, and cooling of the forehead.

In treating migraine, Schultz and Luthe reported that, through the use of autogenic training exercises, the majority of their patients had fewer and less intense headaches. A number of patients reported a cure after several months of practice and learned to interrupt the onset of an attack by starting autogenic exercises as soon as prodromal symptoms appeared.

Biofeedback training, a recently developed technique, holds promise of accelerating psychosomatic self-regulation. This technique, when combined with autogenic phrases, is called autogenic feedback training. It uses visual and auditory devices to show the subject what is happening to normally unconscious bodily functions as he or she attempts to influence them by use of mental, emotional, and somatic visualizations. One experimental physiological function was increasing the blood flow in the hands as an index of the voluntary control of the autonomic nervous system. Work in our laboratory has shown that skin temperature in the hands is directly related to blood flow in the hands [19].

The possibility of using autogenic feedback training for migraine patients was suggested by the experience of a research subject who, during the spontaneous recovery from a migraine attack, demonstrated considerable flushing in her hands with an accompanying ten-degree rise in two minutes. Knowledge of this event quickly spread through the laboratory and prompted two migraineurs to volunteer for training in hand-temperature control. One volunteer was wholly successful; the other had a partially beneficial result. On the basis of this experience, it seemed useful to conduct further study with headache patients in a clinical setting.

EXPERIENCE WITH PSYCHOSOMATIC SELF-REGULATION IN MIGRAINE TREATMENT

Gellhorn [20] discussed the concept of central nervous system tuning and thoroughly reviewed the literature on conditioning of the central nervous system. His article provides a strong rationale for using cortical processes to reverse an excitatory state of subcortical structures. Thus, he provides a functional framework of how mind and body work together and also a conceptual framework for the term "psychosomatic."

Unfortunately, this term has been thought to be primarily in the domain of the psychiatrist, with the psychoanalyst as the ultimate authority. This attitude has consequently narrowed medical interest in the concept. Social conditions (sociopsychosomatic) are another element of a triad that could be added but will not be discussed because of my desire to concentrate on the relationship of mind and body. They are connected by a nervous-system and metabolic network dominated by the hypothalamic-pituitary hormonal axis.

Alterations in physiological function often accompany changes in a person's mental status, and this change often involves an interpretation of external events which may be adaptive or maladaptive. So-called stress may be associated with pleasant or unpleasant events, and a migraine attack is precipitated under both conditions.

The model of Gaader (Figure 1) is helpful in conceptualizing the interrelationships between mind, body, and environment. In this model there is a reciprocal relationship between the central processor and all other portions of the body. Each of the heavy lines represents a biofeedback system. No. 1 completes a loop between the cortical and subcortical

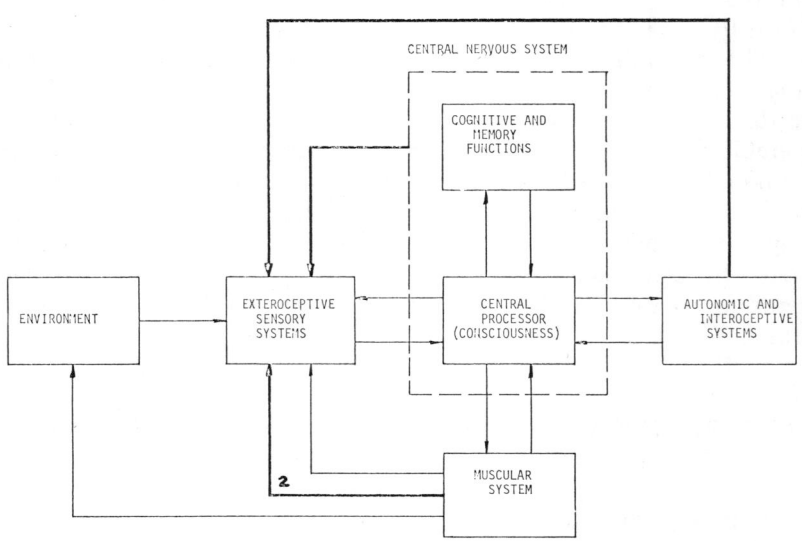

Figure 1. *Psychophysiological feedback. (Reprinted with permission from Gaader KR and Montgomery PS: Clinical Biofeedback, a Procedural Manual, 24. Baltimore, Williams & Wilkins, 1977.)*

portions of the central nervous system and its sensory component. No. 2 deals with the influence of the muscular system on the sensory system. It should be noted also that the only way an organism affects the environment is through the muscular system. No. 3 represents the specific feedback of information concerned with internal functioning. An example of such feedback is the use of skin temperature to give knowledge of the status of the hand vasculature. Previous work in our laboratories has shown that hand temperature is a good reflector of the vasomotor tone of the hand blood vessels, with an increase in temperature inversely proportional to vasomotor tone [19, 20]. Our treatment of migraine with the use of autogenic feedback training to increase blood flow into the hands began in 1969, and the final report of our preliminary studies was published in 1975 [21, 22, 23].

The pilot work was carried out over a five-and-a-half year period. During this time 110 migraine subjects entered the project and 36 dropped out before completing 270 days of training and follow-up. The 74 who completed training and follow-up were evaluated for the percentage of reduction in headache activity in a later period as compared to an earlier period of the project. The later period of comparison was after the graduates completed 181 to 270 days of post-training. The earlier period was different for two sub-groups of the graduates. For 54 graduates, this period was 90 days before training began; for the remaining 20 graduates it was 0 to 90 days after the start of training. In looking at the data for a follow-up study two years after the pilot study, a different distribution of the graduates in the five groups of headache improvement was obtained (Table 1). The change in the distribution curves does not significantly

Table 1

Follow-up Study of Thermal-Training Graduates

Percentage Reduction in Headache Activity	Categories of Improvement	Number of Subjects in Each Category	
		New	Old
0–9	none	12	12
10–25	slight	11	7
26–50	moderate	16	22
51–75	good	20	16
76–100	very good	15	17
	Total number completing 270 days of training and follow-up	74	74

alter the evidence suggesting possible usefulness of thermal training in controlling migraine headaches.

To date, published long-term assessments of biofeedback success are few and they are scattered throughout the medical and psychological literature. In early 1975 we did a follow-up on the 110 subjects in the preliminary study [24]. The 74 who had completed the pilot project (henceforth called graduates) had a response rate of 76 percent, or 56 of the 74. This was accomplished by two mailings of a questionnaire and subsequent telephone calls. Belatedly, we decided to check on the 36 who had not completed the study (henceforth known as dropouts), but only 12 could be reached.

Nonrespondents were found to be similar in most respects to respondents in both the graduate and dropout groups; in particular, the distribution of success in controlling headaches for respondents and nonrespondents in both groups was not significantly different (Table 2).

A significant difference in the pattern of practice was found, with graduate respondents practicing more routinely than dropout respondents. Sixty-six percent of the graduate respondents practiced once a week to several times a day, while 56 percent of the dropout respondents usually practiced only when they felt tension or an impending headache. In the graduate respondent group, 7.5 percent had an increase in headache frequency, 77.4 percent had a decrease, and 15.1 percent showed no change. In comparison, no one in the dropout respondent group had an increase in headache frequency, while 88.9 percent had a decrease, and 11.1 percent did not change.

Of the graduates, 3.8 percent did not respond to the question regarding headache frequency, 73.6 percent showed a decrease in headache intensity, 17 percent remained the same, and 5.7 percent had an increase.

Table 2

Comparison of Graduate and Dropout Groups

1. Frequency of practice	$\chi^2 = 34.3$, df $= 7$; $p < 0.0005$
2. Decrease in headache frequency	$\chi^2 = 0.9$, df $= 2$; N.S.
3. Decrease in headache intensity	$\chi^2 = 7.6$, df $= 3$; $p < 0.10$
4. Decrease in headache duration	$\chi^2 = 13.5$. df $= 3$; $p < 0.005$
5. Decrease in medication usage	$\chi^2 = 16.6$, df $= 3$; $p < 0.001$

For headache intensity in the dropout group, 11.1 percent had an increase, 33.3 percent reported a decrease, and 55.6 percent remained the same.

In the graduate group, 73.6 percent demonstrated a drop in headache duration, 1.9 percent had an increase, 18.9 percent remained the same, and 8.7 percent did not answer. Of the dropouts, 22.2 percent reported a decrease in headache duration and 77.8 percent did not change.

In regard to medication usage, the graduate group had 71.7 percent with a decrease, 9.4 percent with an increase, 15.1 percent with no change, and 3.8 percent who did not answer. In contrast, the dropout group had 22.2 percent with a decrease and 77.8 percent who remained the same.

Respondents in both groups showed similar decreases in headache frequency, suggesting that both groups got something out of participating in the project. The difference between the two groups for headache intensity was only of borderline significance. The difference between frequency of practice is striking, with the graduate respondents doing thermal training much more and showing very significant decreases in headache duration and medication usage. Thus, as long as two years after conclusion of the pilot study, the graduate respondents did maintain their success in controlling their migraine headaches, allowing marked reduction in their use of medication.

Because the results of our follow-up study show a sustained improvement in a substantial number of migraineurs who used thermal training, controlled studies assume more importance in determining whether or not thermal training has a specific effect in managing migraine attacks.

Taub and Emurian [25] taught 19 of 20 consecutive subjects to learn autoregulatory control of hand skin temperature and found that, as the subjects' mastery increased, the response became more localized to the trained portion of the body. At this point transfer of control to other portions of the body was readily accomplished and regulation in the new area was also specific. During transfer testing, two subjects were asked to increase their forehead temperature. After they raised their temperature three to four degrees, severe headaches of quick onset developed. Wickramasekera [26] described two migraineurs who did not respond to forehead EMG feedback training but later did respond to increasing blood flow in the hands. Koppman et al. [27], working with voluntary regulation of the temporal artery caliber in ten migraine subjects, showed that patients were able to regulate their temporal arteries and control their migraine headaches. Budzynski et al. have had reasonable success in controlling tension headaches by using EMG feedback training of the frontalis muscle [28]. This biofeedback technique had little success in controlling migraine headaches, but increasing blood flow in the hands worked well [29].

Two previous studies of accelerated training procedures demonstrated similar, yet differing, results. Diamond and Franklin [30] found that this approach led to improvement while subjects were in training; Pearse and her colleagues [31] showed that improvement in headache could be maintained by headache patients after they left training. In contrast, the former authors found substantial problems in subjects after they left the supportive environment of the clinic.

Mitch et al. [32] showed improvement in 11 of 15 migrainous subjects over a three-month period of training with autogenic phrases and continuous temperature feedback. Sheridan et al. [33] compared 40 subjects' voluntary control of hand-warming under four conditions: control, autogenic biofeedback, autogenic phrases alone, and biofeedback alone. They concluded that autogenic phrases alone might provide a simpler effective therapy for disorders currently treated with autogenic biofeedback and biofeedback alone. Blanchard et al. [34], in a study of 30 migraineurs, compared temperature feedback with autogenic training, progressive relaxation, and a control group. All groups showed a significant decrease in headache frequency, while the biofeedback and relaxation groups did not differ on any dependent measure. Turin and Johnson [35] found that warming was more effective than cooling of the hands in reducing seven migrainous subjects' headaches. Medina et al. [36] reported that 13 of 17 migraineurs improved significantly for an average of 14.2 months after training, initially with EMG from frontalis area and subsequently with increasing hand blood flow. Benson et al. [37] showed that in 17 patients the relaxation response from practicing transcendental meditation had limited usefulness in decreasing migraine and cluster headaches.

For childhood migraine, Diamond and Franklin [38] reported the usefulness of combining EMG feedback and thermal training. Their 32 subjects' ages ranged from 9 to 18. Reading and Mohr [39] showed statistically and clinically significant improvement in several indices of migraine activity in six subjects who used biofeedback for regulation of hand temperature to control migraine headaches.

Drury et al. [40], using the multiple baseline technique, showed that the treatment package of instructions aimed at generating favorable therapeutic expectations, and the use of autogenic phrases and fingertip temperature feedback in relaxation training, had an impact on migraine headaches.

The literature to date presents a confusing array of observations about the usefulness of thermal training to control migraine headache. A definitive study is needed to search for a specific effect of thermal training in migraine. We are in the process of examining data from our controlled clinical outcome study, which evaluates this question.

INTEGRATION OF PSYCHOSOMATIC SELF-REGULATION INTO MEDICALLY RECOGNIZED THERAPIES

Our clinical experience suggests that psychosomatic self-regulation may be used as a substitute for medications in treating patients for migraine headaches, but there are limitations to its efficacy. If pain builds up so rapidly that a patient is overwhelmed by it, psychosomatic self-regulation will not work. It is also not helpful when the patient has reached the stage at which nausea and vomiting occur. In both of these situations the addition of medications to the self-regulation technique is helpful. Headaches that awaken a patient from sleep are difficult to control, and, here too, medications are needed.

If a patient fails to learn to increase the blood flow in his hands, the failure cannot be ascribed to the technique. Many patients lack the motivation to learn this skill. At times prolonged work with a patient leads nowhere, and in these cases psychiatric consultation may help to uncover feelings that prevent a patient from applying the technique effectively.

These are some situations in which integration of medically recognized therapies provides additional benefit over selective use of any one of the therapies.

SUMMARY

A framework was developed to help those interested in psychosomatic self-regulation learn why it might help to control migraine headache. The accuracy of this hypothesis will become evident as we learn more about the physiology and biochemistry of migraine and brain function. Clinical evidence for the usefulness of this tool in migraine has far outstripped our knowledge of these basic issues. From my clinical experience, psychosomatic self-regulation works best when it is used in relationship with other time-proven therapies.

REFERENCES

1. Graham JR, Wolff HG: The mechanism of the migraine headache and the action of ergotamine tartrate. *Arch Neurol Psychiatry* 39:737, 1938.
2. Pickering GW, Hess W: Observations on the mechanism of headache produced by histamine. *Clinical Science* 51:77, 1933.
3. Clark D, Hough W, Wolff HG: Experimental studies on headache observations on histamine headaches. *Archives of Medrology and Psychiatry* 23:140, 1932.
4. Schumacher GA, Wolff HG: Experimental studies of headache. *Archives of Medrology and Psychiatry* 45:199, 1941.
5. Dukes HT, Vieth RG: Cerebral arteriography during migraine prodrome and headache. *Neurology* 14:636, 1964.
6. Edmeads J: Vascular headaches and the cranial circulation—another look. *Headache* 19:127–130, 1979.
7. Wolff GH: *Headache and Other Head Pain*, 2nd Ed. New York, Oxford University Press, 1963.
8. Sicuteri F: Vasoneuroreactive substances and their implications in vascular pain, in Friedman AP (ed): *Research and Clinical Studies of Headache*. Baltimore, Williams & Wilkins, 1967.
9. Lance JW, Anthony M, Hinterberger H: The control of cranial arteries by humoral mechanism and its relation to the migraine syndrome. *Headache* 7:93–102, 1967.
10. Pearce J: *Migraine: Clinical Features, Mechanisms and Management*. Springfield, Illinois, Thomas, 1969.
11. Herberg LJ: The hypothalamus and the aetiology of migraine, in Smith R (ed): *Background to Migraine*. London, Heineman, 1967.
12. Rao LS, Pearce J: Hypothalamic-pituitary-adrenal axis studies in studies with special reference to insulin sensitivity. *Brain* 94:289–298, 1971.
13. Herberg LJ: Migraine and the locus coeruleus. *Migraine News* 36:1–4, 1978.
14. Kentsmith D, Strider F, Copenhauer J, Jacques D: Effects of biofeedback upon suppression of migraine symptoms and plasma dopamine-β-hydroxylase activity. *Headache* 16:173–177, 1976.
15. Mathew RJ, Ho BT, Kralik P, Claghorn JL: Biochemical basis for biofeedback treatment of migraine: A hypothesis. *Headache* 19:290–293, 1979.
16. Miller ME: Learning of visceral and glandular responses. *Science* 163:434–445, 1969.
17. Green EE, Ferguson DW, Green AM, Walters ED: *Preliminary Report on Voluntary Controls Project: Swami Rama*. The Menninger Foundation, June, 1970.
18. Schultz JH, Luthe W: *Autogenic Therapy* (Volume I). New York, Grune & Stratton, 1969.
19. Sargent JD, Green EE, Walters ED: The use of autogenic feedback training in a pilot study of migraine and tension headaches. *Headache* 12:120–124, 1972.
20. Gellhorn E: Central nervous system tuning and its implications for neuropsychiatry. *J Nerv Ment Dis* 147:148–162, 1968.

21. Sargent JD, Green EE, Walters ED: Preliminary report on the use of autogenous feedback training in the treatment of migraine and tension headaches. *Psychosom Med* 35:129–135, 1972.
22. Sargent JD, Green EE, Walters ED: Psychosomatic self-regulation of migraine and tension headaches. *Seminars in Psychiatry* 5:415–428, 1973.
23. Sargent JD, Taylor J, Coyne L, Thetford P, Walters ED, Segerson J: Progress report: Autogenic feedback in migraine headaches. *J Kans Med Soc* 76:266–267, 1975.
24. Solbach P, Sargent JD: A follow-up evaluation of the Menninger pilot migraine headache study using thermal training. *Headache* 17:198–202, 1977.
25. Taub E, Emurian CS: Feedback aided self-regulation of skin temperature with a single feedback locus: 1. Acquisition and reversal training. *Biofeedback Self Regul* 1:147–168, 1976.
26. Wickramasekera IE: Temperature feedback for the control of migraine. *Journal of Behavior Therapy and Experimental Psychiatry* 4:343–345, 1973.
27. Koppman JW, McDonald RD, Kunzel MG: Voluntary regulation of temporal artery diameter by migraine patients. *Headache* 14:133–137.
28. Budzynski T, Stoyva J, Adler C: Feedback-induced relaxation: Application to tension headache. *Journal of Behavioral Therapy and Experimental Psychiatry* 1:205–211, 1970.
29. Budzynski T: Biofeedback procedures in the clinic. *Seminars in Psychiatry* 5:540, 1973.
30. Diamond S, Franklin M: Intensive biofeedback therapy in the treatment of headache. Presented to Biofeedback Research Society Sixth Annual Meeting, Monterey, Cal., 1975.
31. Pearse B, Sargent J, Walters D, Meer M: Exploratory observations of the use of an intensive autogenic biofeedback training (IAFT) procedure in a follow-up study of out-of-town patients having migraine and/or tension headaches. Presented to Biofeedback Research Society Sixth Annual Meeting, Monterey, Cal., 1975.
32. Mitch P, McGrady A, Iannone A: Autogenic feedback training in migraine: A treatment report. *Headache* 15:267–270, 1976.
33. Sheridan C, Boehm M, Ward L, Justensen D: Autogenic-biofeedback, autogenic phrases, and biofeedback compared. Presented to Biofeedback Research Society Seventh Annual Meeting, Colorado Springs, 1976.
34. Blanchard E, Theobald DE, Williamson MS, Silver BV, Brown DA: Temperature biofeedback in the treatment of migraine headache—a controlled evaluation. *Arch Gen Psychiatry* 35:581–588, 1978.
35. Turin A, Johnson W: Biofeedback therapy for migraine headaches. *Arch Gen Psychiatry* 33:517–519, 1975.
36. Medina J, Diamond S, Franklin M: Biofeedback therapy for migraine. *Headache* 16:115–118, 1976.
37. Benson H, Klemchuk H, Graham J: The usefulness of the relaxation response in the therapy of headache. *Headache* 14:49–52, 1974.
38. Diamond S, Franklin M: Biofeedback—choice of treatment in childhood migraine.

Presented to Biofeedback Research Society Seventh Annual Meeting, Colorado Springs, 1976.
39. Reading C, Mohr P: Biofeedback control of migraine: A pilot study. *Br J Soc Clin Psychol* 15:429–433, 1976.
40. Drury RL, Derisi WJ, Liberman RP: Temperature biofeedback treatment for migraine headaches: A controlled multiple baseline study. *Headache* 19:278–284, 1979.

Chapter 7
Cerebral Blood Flow and Headache Activity in Normal Volunteers and Migraineurs Trained in Skin Temperature Self-Regulation

JOHN W. LARGEN, JR., PH.D.
ROY J. MATHEW, M.D.

MIGRAINE HEADACHE

Since the advent of biofeedback methodology in the early 1960s, subsequent research and clinical applications in the 1970s have shown biofeedback to be an effective behavioral treatment tool for a host of stress-related disorders. One of the most consistent and successful applications of biofeedback has been in the management of migraine headache.

Vascular headache of the migraine type is a common neurologic disorder characterized by recurrent attacks of headache which vary widely in frequency, severity, and duration [1]. The headaches are generally unilateral in onset, of a throbbing character, and may be associated with any subset of the following: photophobia, phonophobia, anorexia, constipation, diarrhea, nausea, and occasional vomiting [2–4].

Migraine headache traditionally has been treated pharmacologically (symptomatic and prophylactic) and to some extent with psychologic methods (including psychotherapy, hypnosis, relaxation training, and behavioral therapy). Given the difficulties often encountered with headache medications (nonresponsivenes, habituation, adverse side effects, and addiction), the advent of an effective nonpharmacological treatment has generated considerable interest.

This chapter will focus primarily upon peripheral skin temperature control and its application to the management of migraine headache. Several physiologic modalities amenable to biofeedback training have been applied to the management of migraine headache including self-regulation of peripheral skin temperature and extracranial vasomotor response, electromyography (EMG), and electroencephalography (EEG). However, skin temperature control and extracranial vasomotor self-regulation have produced the most consistent results [5].

The serendipitous discovery by Sargent and co-workers that hand-warming learned via biofeedback may be an effective behavioral technique in migraine management [6-8] ushered in a substantial number of studies from independent laboratories that confirmed the efficacy of the procedure. Recently these studies have been well summarized by Price [9], Ray et al. [5], and Diamond et al. [10] who wrote the task force report on the biofeedback treatment of vascular headache commissioned by the Biofeedback Society of America (update included in this volume). Though not without criticism, the consensus of these reviews is that skin temperature self-regulation (either alone or in conjunction with relaxation techniques) may reduce the frequency, severity, and duration of migraine headache in a substantial proportion of headache sufferers. The board of directors of the American Association for the Study of Headache recently endorsed biofeedback therapy as a valid form of treatment for headache [11].

Research in biofeedback and migraine has been criticized [5, 9]. Notably absent, in the early research in particular, were adequately designed studies with sufficient baseline, follow-up, and statistical treatment of the data [12]. The treatment protocols often included mixed factors, such as suggestion and relaxation in addition to biofeedback training. There was often a lack of control groups to assess placebo effects [12], and there was little evidence that hand-warming techniques produced any contribution over and above that of traditional relaxation techniques [13]. Taub [14] pointed out the absence of reported data on the proportion of subjects who attained skin temperature control and the degree of control achieved. Even fewer studies have attempted to relate these changes to alterations in migraine activity. Finally, the physiologic rationale for using skin temperature self-regulation in the management of migraine has not been articulated clearly, nor has the role of nonspecific (nontemperature) factors been adequately assessed [5]. In reviewing

CEREBRAL BLOOD FLOW AND HEADACHE ACTIVITY 93

abstracts pertaining to hand-warming and migraine, one is apt to find studies that hypothesize opposite effects in cephalic blood flow hemodynamics, without adequate consideration of the headache phase involved or whether the effects occur intra- or extracranially.

This chapter is mainly an annotated summary of two pilot studies conducted in the Psychosomatic Research Laboratory of the Texas Research Institute of Mental Sciences, in collaboration with the Regional Cerebral Blood Flow Laboratory, Department of Neurology, Baylor College of Medicine. Detailed descriptions of these studies and their findings are in previously published reports [15–17].

A major goal in the investigations was to define the relationship between the skin temperature component in the hand-warming procedure and the therapeutic gains derived in migraine management.

A second issue was to clarify the mechanism involved: how a factor as seemingly unrelated as warming hands could influence migraine activity. At present, theories to account for the therapeutic gains in migraine management remain unclear and are somewhat simplistic, though they provide valuable heuristic models around which hypotheses may be constructed and tested. The theoretical notions may be clarified if the relationship betwen changes in cerebral blood flow and skin temperature self-control can be delineated.

The data were evaluated at three levels of analysis: behavioral (headache activity), physiologic (regional cerebral blood flow), and the interactions of the two.

The present studies were designed to answer the following questions:

> Do hand-warming and hand-cooling differentially affect migraine activity?
>
> What role do temperature-specific and nonspecific factors play in the management of migraine headache?
>
> Does hand-warming have both symptomatic and prophylactic effects on migraine headache activity?
>
> Is skin temperature self-control associated with changes in regional cerebral blood flow?
>
> In terms of regional cerebral blood flow changes, do normal volunteers differ from migraineurs when exposed to the identical paradigm?
>
> Do hand-warming and hand-cooling produce different patterns of regional cerebral blood flow?
>
> What mechanisms are suggested to account for the successful application of hand-warming techniques to migraine headache?

What interactions are there between skin temperature control and regional cerebral blood flow, skin temperature control and headache activity, and regional cerebral blood flow and headache activity?

The basic paradigm was as follows: Two groups of normal volunteers and migraineurs were each randomly divided into a "hand-warming" group and "hand-cooling" group and trained in skin temperature self-regulation. Thus the difference between the groups in terms of specific temperature components was maximized, while nonspecific components were held constant. Following biofeedback training, all subjects were given two measurements of regional cerebral blood flow: one measure during a steady-state, resting condition and a second measure while the subjects were attempting to regulate their skin temperature. Hand-warmers were compared to hand-coolers, and normals compared to migraineurs in terms of direction and pattern of associated regional cerebral blood flow changes. In the migraine group, hand-warmers were also compared to hand-coolers in terms of pretraining versus post-training headache activity.

If temperature-specific factors represented the dominant components in migraine management, then hand-warming groups and hand-cooling groups would be expected to exhibit differential changes in headache activity and regional cerebral blood flow. If nonspecific effects were the major active components, then both temperature groups would be expected to demonstrate similar patterns of change in terms of headache activity and regional cerebral blood flow.

SUBJECT CHARACTERISTICS

Normal Group

Twelve right-handed women were selected from volunteers who responded to posted advertisements requesting volunteers for a biofeedback experiment. Mean age was 33.2 years (range = 22 to 37 years). Excluded were those with migraine, hypertension, pregnancy, those taking vasoactive or sympathomimetic drugs, or those manifesting any serious psychiatric disorders.

Migraine Group

Migraine volunteers were also sought via posted advertisements, though many were referred by physicians. Selected were 13 female migraineurs who were strongly right-handed (Harris Test of Lateral Dominance) and had a mean age of 38.1 years (range = 27 to 52 years). Of particular significance was the careful selection of exclusively "textbook" cases of classic and common migraine. Such a task proved to be a difficult endeavor as witnessed by the selection of only 13 patients from a pool of more than 100 migraine volunteers. All diagnoses were established by neurologists following a complete medical history and neurologic evaluation including at least three of the following: skull x-ray, electroencephalogram, brain scan, cranial tomography (CT scan), pneumoencephalogram, and regional cerebral blood flow measurement.

Migraine headache was operationally defined as an intermittent headache of sufficient severity to impair the patient's daily functioning significantly. Patients selected had a minimum of two migraine headaches per month in addition to at least three of the following:

1. Predominantly unilateral head pain
2. Pulsating quality of pain
3. Nausea and/or vomiting
4. Photophobia/phonophobia
5. Positive family history
6. Visual aura or other transitory neurological disturbance preceding and possibly lasting into the headache phase

Excluded were patients who reported any indication of mixed migraine headache or muscle-contraction headache, defined as headaches occurring almost daily, of a mild to severe nature, usually bilateral, characterized by band-like pressure across the forehead, and a dull nonthrobbing ache. Of the subjects who completed the study, eight had been diagnosed as having common migraine and three as having classic migraine. Mean frequency of headache was 3.3 to 4.0 headaches per month with a median duration of 15 hours each. Average age of onset was age 23 with a headache history of about 15 years. There were no remarkable features in the patients' psychiatric or medical histories. None were taking prophylactic medications during the study, and their headaches were managed with ergot compounds and/or analgesics with varying degrees of success.

PROCEDURES AND METHODS

With random division of the volunteers and migraine patients into a hand-warming and hand-cooling group, care was taken to match the migraine groups for classification of headache so that classic and common migraine patients were represented equally in each temperature group.

Data for five subjects were excluded because the subjects either dropped out or did not comply with the study protocol. Subjects who completed the study were four normal hand-warmers, five normal hand-coolers, six migraine hand-warmers, and five migraine hand-coolers. The two temperature groups showed no significant pretraining differences in age, frequency, severity, or duration of migraine headaches.

Headache Records

Headache activity was carefully recorded for five weeks before biofeedback training, during training, and for a minimum of five weeks afterward on record sheets provided by the experimenters [18, 19]. Information concerning the distribution of head pain was collected with the help of a coded fascimile of left and right sides of the head. The record also contained a grid to indicate headache intensity along the horizontal axis and time and duration of occurrence along the vertical axis, so that subject ratings of headache intensity could be plotted for each waking hour of headache. Headache intensity was rated on a six-point scale containing descriptive definitions of intensity level. Medication type and dosage were also recorded, as was the patient's subjective estimate of success in self-regulating temperature and effect on the headache.

Seven headache variables were derived: two medication indices, two duration indices, two severity indices, and headache frequency.

Biofeedback Training

Normal and migraine subjects were extensively trained in the self-regulation of skin temperature for five weeks in an average of three sessions per week.

Each 35-minute session consisted of a 15-minute stabilization period and a 20-minute training period during which the subject received biofeedback. The first two training sessions were devoted to acquisition of relaxation skills via auditory feedback of forehead EMG activity, supplemented by taped instructions in progressive relaxation [20]. The third and subsequent sessions concentrated on the training of skin temperature control. After the 15-minute stabilization period, patients received auditory feedback over earphones; feedback consisted of a steady pulsating tone whose pitch was directly proportional to skin temperature of the patient's right middle finger. Forehead EMG was integrated over five-minute periods, and absolute skin temperature was recorded at one-minute intervals throughout the session.

The experimenter maintained an enthusiastic, supportive, and empathetic rapport with patients and encouraged them to develop their own strategies for skin temperature control. The critical value of practicing relaxation and skin temperature control at home was emphasized, and patients were instructed to practice twice a day for 15 minutes. Migraine patients were instructed to begin their temperature control strategies at the first indication of a migraine headache.

^{133}Xenon Inhalation Method

After completing biofeedback training, each patient was given two measures of regional cerebral blood flow (rCBF) separated by a 30-minute resting interval. One measurement was taken while the subject relaxed comfortably in a steady-state condition with eyes closed, in a darkened room with silence maintained. A second measurement was taken while subjects attempted to alter their skin temperature in the trained direction with biofeedback.

Immediately before both measurements, a relaxation tape was played to facilitate relaxation. The order of relaxation and biofeedback runs was counterbalanced within each temperature group to control for "order" effects. None of the subjects had suffered a migraine headache within three days before the rCBF measurements.

Regional cerebral blood flow was measured by the noninvasive ^{133}Xenon inhalation technique using the measurement and analysis principles of Obrist and co-workers [21, 22] and later modified by Meyer and associates [23–25]. (Detailed description of procedure in chapter 1, this volume.)

BEHAVIORAL LEVEL OF ANALYSIS: HEADACHE ACTIVITY

Is there a difference in headache activity between patients trained to warm and cool their hands?

This issue has important implications for the theoretical understanding of mechanism as well as practical application. Is the skin temperature factor itself a key component in alleviating migraine headache? The question is whether migraine headache responds primarily to temperature-specific or nonspecific effects.

A review of the literature provides the background for an understanding of the issues involved. Since the initial studies by Sargent and co-workers [6–8] linking skin temperature self-regulation and successful migraine mitigation, research and clinical evidence has accumulated which support the utility of hand-warming techniques.

Earlier reports pointed to a specific skin temperature factor as the most active component in the behavioral management of migraine. Observations of a more anecdotal nature suggested that migraine headache responded preferentially to skin temperature biofeedback alone or skin temperature control in combination with various relaxation procedures including EMG feedback-assisted relaxation [6, 19, 26, 27]. Turin and Johnson [28] demonstrated that migraine patients trained to warm their hands showed substantial clinical improvement in all dependent variables measured, while the hand-coolers showed either no change or an exacerbation of headache activity. When given subsequent training in hand-warming, these patients' headaches improved.

Thus the combined observations of these early studies led to the tacit acceptance of a functional relationship between skin temperature self-regulation and migraine headache activity, thereby implying a specific temperature effect.

In contrast, more recent studies have cast doubt on this interpretation and have supported nonspecific variables as the most significant components. Andreychuk and Skriver [29] compared three treatment strategies in 13 migraine patients: biofeedback-assisted hand-warming, biofeedback-assisted alpha enhancement, and self-hypnosis. Using a headache index based on duration and intensity, all three groups showed significant reductions in headache rate with no significant differences between the groups. In a study by Bakal and Kaganov [18], EMG biofeedback was found to be effective in producing significantly reduced headache scores in both migraine and tension headache patients. Mullinix et al. [30] trained an experimental migraine group in a hand-warming task, using true "contingent" auditory feedback of their skin temperature performance while a control group received noncontingent "false" feedback. Compared to the control group, the contingent feedback group learned to increase their skin temperature significantly. Both groups showed similar improvement in headache activity and medication required. Neither Mullinix and co-workers [30] nor Werbach and Sandweiss [31] found significant correlations between the degree of skin temperature change and headache improvement.

In a control-group outcome evaluation of biofeedback and migraine, Blanchard et al. [32] compared a group trained in skin temperature biofeedback plus autogenic relaxation procedures, a group trained in progressive relaxation, and a control group of patients on the waiting list. Following training all three groups demonstrated significant decline in headache frequency. Both treatment groups showed significant improvement in total headache activity, duration of headache, peak headache intensity, and medication consumption compared to the controls who showed no such changes. In a later one-year follow-up study [33] there continued to be a maintenance of the beneficial effects with no difference between the progressive relaxation and temperature biofeedback groups, with the exception of medication consumption in which the relaxation group showed greater continued improvement. The importance of daily home practice, expectation of success, and application of learned strategies at the onset of a migraine headache were emphasized in the majority of studies reviewed above.

The implied conclusion from the later studies is that peripheral skin temperature training is merely one of several avenues to success, and that the therapeutic gains observed in the biofeedback treatment of migraine results from some factor or factors shared by the various treatment approaches, independent of skin temperature self-control.

In the present study, post-training headache data were compared to pre-training data for migraineurs trained to warm or cool their hands. Seven headache variables were derived from individual headache data recorded by each of the patients in the two groups. "Per month" variables represented totals which were standardized to a 30-day recording period. "Per headache" data were derived by dividing the nonstandardized totals by the number of headaches.

The grouped headache variables are displayed in Figure 1. The derived indices were as follows:

Analgesic Units

Analgesic units were based upon the "relative potency scale" developed by Coyne et al. [34]. The assigned weight for a given analgesic was multiplied by its dosage, thereby yielding "analgesic units" for a given headache.

Duration

The significance of dual indices of headache activity is more easily demonstrated with duration. For example, if a migraineur typically experienced two 10-hour headaches per month and then, after treatment, experienced ten 2-hour headaches per month, it would be equally important to know that, in both cases, the total number of headache hours per month was 20 and had not changed. But the mean hours per headache had changed from 10 to 2. Similarly, the analogy applies to other dual indices.

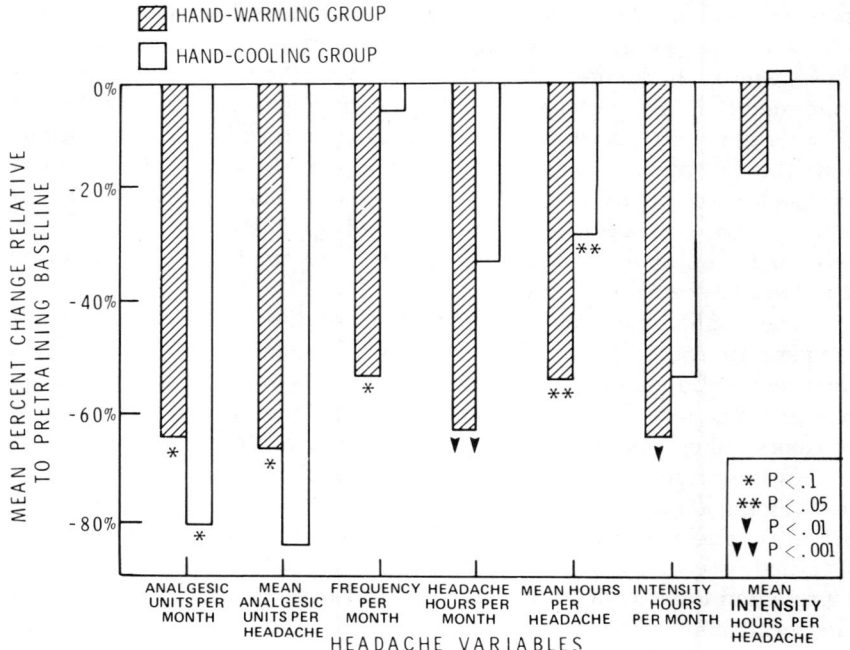

Figure 1. Mean percentage of change in headache variables after biofeedback training. A negative percentage indicates lessening or improvement of symptom.

Severity

Intensity hours were derived by multiplying the number of headache hours at a given intensity by that intensity score and then summated for each headache.

Figure 1 suggests that the active components of the treatment package are primarily nonspecific in nature with some indication of a temperature-specific effect as well, depending upon the symptom examined.

Nonspecific Effects

Regardless of the direction of skin temperature control, both groups improved substantially in quantity/quality of medication consumed on a monthly basis, medication per headache, number of headache hours per month, mean number of hours per headache, and total severity of headache per month. These data suggest that nonspecific factors independent of the direction of skin temperature control were largely responsible for the improvements in headache activity.

Individual Variability

Figure 1 represents the grouped headache data. However, individual patterns of symptom change revealed substantial variability. Had a single global headache index been used as the prime dependent variable, subjects in both temperature groups would have shown improvement. The present study underscores the importance of fractionalizing the data into the key headache components, so that patterns of change may be seen. The variability extended not only to the patterns of change but the magnitude of change as well. Thus subjects displayed different topographies of change in headache activity in association with skin temperature control. Certain subjects showed across-the-board improvement of large magnitude in all headache variables, while others demonstrated improvement in a few symptoms with either no change or a slight worsening in other variables. The individual differences may result from a number of variables: steadiness of home practice, initial level of individual headache component, learning ability, or individual response specificity [35], among others.

Temperature-Specific Effects

Figure 1 reveals a tendency toward divergence in two symptoms: headache frequency and, to a lesser extent, mean intensity hours per headache. For headache frequency, $5/6$ or 83 percent of the patients trained to warm their hands showed an improvement, compared to $4/5$ or 80 percent of the hand-coolers who exhibited either no change or an exacerbation of headache frequency. Four of six hand-warmers showed a mild to marked improvement in mean intensity hours per headache, while only one hand-cooler demonstrated an improvement in this variable. With the exception of the medication indices, the hand-warming group generally showed improvements of greater magnitude than the hand-cooling group in other headache indices. Thus these data demonstrate a superiority of hand-warming over hand-cooling.

These data are somewhat compatible with the headache frequency data of Turin and Johnson [28] but differ in terms of their medication measures which also showed divergent trends.

The present results were also compatible with a double-blind study by Kewman and Roberts [36] who compared one group of migraineurs trained in hand-warming, a group trained in hand-cooling, and a third who received no treatment. When the data were analyzed according to a learning criterion irrespective of the original group assignment, the combined groups showed a significant improvement in the duration of headache, amount of impairment, and the amount of medication. In relation to the group who learned to decrease their skin temperature, however, the other groups combined showed significant improvement in frequency of migraine, number of symptoms per week, minutes of headache per week, and medication per week, suggesting a treatment effect. The authors interpreted their overall results as being mediated largely by nonspecific variables.

In summary, the behavioral data suggest that the active components of hand-warming consist of a mixed package of nonspecific factors, which represent the most salient effects and, to a lesser extent, temperature-specific effects.

What is the relationship between skin temperature and headache variables?

Silver and Blanchard [37] reviewed studies in which biofeedback techniques had been applied to psychophysiological and "stress-related" disorders. These authors posed the question, "Are the machines really necessary?" The question implies two components: first, whether the machines are necessary to learn the appropriate physiological response and second, whether the learned response is related to changes in the symptoms. Budzynski [38] has pointed to four possible outcomes of biofeedback applications to headache: (a) Response learned, headache disappears; (b) response learned, no change in headache; (c) response not learned, headache disappears; and (d) response not learned, no change in headache. Outcomes a and d suggest some potential relationship between learned physiological response and clinical symptoms. Outcomes b and c suggest little relationship but implicate other nonspecific factors.

In our study, all migraine subjects achieved at least moderate control of skin temperature in the trained direction. There was, however, substantial between-subject and between-session variability in the magnitude and consistency of that control. In the hand-warming group, individual peak warming trends in the final three sessions ranged from 0.61° C to 4.38° C; the peak cooling trends for the hand-cooling group ranged from −.67° C to −4.33° C. As for the relationship to headache symptoms, Table 1 shows correlations between the percentage of change in each headache parameter after training and the mean skin temperature change of the final three training sessions. The correlations are small and nonsignificant, similar to other studies which failed to find significant corre-

Table 1
Correlation between Skin Temperature Self-Regulation (Mean Final 3 Sessions) and Headache Data

	Mean Analgesic Units per Month	Analgesic Units per Headache	Frequency per Month	Headache Hours per Month	Mean Hours per Headache	Mean Intensity Hours per Month	Mean Intensity Hours per Headache
Mean Skin Temperature Change	.28	.33	.02	−.22	−.31	−.26	−.01

lations between degree of skin temperature change and degree of headache improvement [30, 31]. Although Kewman and Roberts [36] found nonsignificant correlations between skin temperature and migraine frequency and duration, they found a correlation of −0.46 between temperature and "the average number of symptoms" and a significant −0.63 correlation with "amount of impairment." The general finding of nonsignificant temperature/headache correlations is not entirely unexpected. Of the few studies which include skin temperature training data, the majority show relatively small learned temperature changes. In addition, there is substantial variability in skin temperature control compared to fairly consistent improvement in headache symptoms. The implication of these data is that the "magnitude" of temperature alteration seems to bear little relationship to migraine headache activity (medication use, headache frequency, duration, intensity) and they provide further evidence for nonspecific factors as the most salient variables in migraine alleviation.

The learned temperature changes recorded in the laboratory are separated in time from the actual application of the temperature-regulating skill outside the laboratory. The question of correlation between skin temperature control and headache activity awaits data gathered on temperature during in vivo applications of attempts to ward off migraine headaches.

Speculation: The key role of relaxation, awareness, and cognitive set

It is of theoretical interest to explore which "nonspecific" factors may play the more significant roles in the reduction of migraine activity.

The nature of migraine does not lend itself easily to clear-cut treatment evaluation. As Friedman [39] has noted, "Few conditions are as unpredictable in their response to treatment as migraine. The clinical picture of a patient with migraine headache may include periods of remission and exacerbation, and such patients may respond to any one of a variety of treatments for a short period of time" (pp. 8–9). Similarly, Miller [13] underscored the "regression to the mean" phenomenon, stressing that patients frequently seek treatment when a fluctuating chronic condition is in a worsened state, and that perceived improvement with treatment may in fact represent a natural fluctuation toward the mean. Miller also commented on the powerful placebo effects of suggestion and experimenter enthusiasm during treatment.

"Nonspecific effects" is a global label suggesting a large number of subject, experimenter, and situational variables often summarized by the term "placebo" [40, 41]. Nonspecific variables include relaxation [20], the self-recording of behaviors [42, 43], and a shift in cognitive set [44, 45]. Inferential evidence suggests that regression to the mean, placebo response, and self-recording of behavior are not the most active mediators of therapeutic gains. Follow-up studies [46–48] indicate that biofeedback treatment benefits may continue up to five years, provided that patients maintain their self-regulatory abilities by practicing. Such data argue against the "regression to the mean" phenomenon and placebo effects' playing a major role, since these variables are known to produce only transitory effects. Furthermore, in migraine studies that include placebo medication as a control, 20 to 30 percent of migraine patients tend to show significant improvement in headache activity [49], compared to 64 to 84 percent of migraine patients who derive significant benefit from biofeedback. With regard to the simple self-recording of migraine behavior, Mitchell and White [50] demonstrated that the self-recording of migraine headaches alone had little effect on reducing headache frequency.

We believe that the relaxation component, sharpening of awareness, and change in cognitive set are the major nonspecific variables in the treatment package.

Relaxation

Relaxation has been shown to be associated with a number of significant physiological changes (including change in oxygen consumption, carbon dioxide elimination, heart rate, respiration, blood lactate, skin resistance, skeletal muscle blood flow, and EEG) [51, 52]. Studies have demonstrated that the continued application of various relaxation techniques to migraine management may result in substantial improvement of headache symptoms.

Luthe [53] reported success in treating migraine patients with autogenic relaxation. Transcendental meditation has also been noted as effective [54]. Hay and Madders [55] described a relaxation treatment program in which 69 of 98 migraine patients showed a decrease in the frequency, severity, or duration of headache attacks. The program involved the training and subsequent application of progressive relaxation, breathing and imagery techniques. Warner and Lance [56] reported successful treatment of 12 migraine patients with muscular and mental relaxation. Eight of the patients showed a greater than 50 percent reduction in headache frequency. Lutker [57] also demonstrated the effectiveness of relaxation techniques in a single case study. Finally, in a direct comparison between thermal biofeedback and progressive relaxation, Blanchard and associates [32] found significant improvement in headache activity in both therapies with no clear-cut advantage for either technique. These data led Silver and Blanchard [37] to conclude that relaxation represented the critical variable in the successful treatment of a number of psychophysiological disorders including migraine, and that relaxation was considered to be the "final common pathway" in treatment.

In a recent review of 85 articles [58], the role of relaxation in biofeedback training was critically examined. The author concluded that either biofeedback or relaxation training alone or in combination was effective in treating migraine headache. However, he noted that "it remains to be discovered whether relaxation methods are more or less effective than other forms of treatment, especially biofeedback procedures; whether these differences are relative to particular disorders; and whether treatment is facilitated when relaxation is combined with biofeedback" (p. 740).

Behavioral and physiological data implicating the skin temperature factor as an important variable may also be interpreted in the context of relaxation. It is possible that volitional increases in skin temperature potentiate the effects of relaxation, while cooling the hands may be physiologically incompatible with or interrupt relaxation.

Relaxation and skin temperature training

To what degree do skin temperature control and relaxation overlap? The two variables would seem to be intimately connected. An analysis of the skin temperature training paradigm reveals a host of overlapping demand characteristics with those of relaxation training. Typically subjects are seated comfortably in a dimly lit room, breathing slowly, with eyes closed. The overlap is even more obvious in the common practice of integrating autogenic relaxation phrases, EMG biofeedback, or progressive relaxation into the temperature training program. Autogenic relaxation phrases alone have been shown to elicit reliable increases in skin temperature following training [59, 60].

Finally, literature on the psychophysiology of emotional states indicates that skin temperature responses may be correlated with varying affective states observed in conjunction with actual interviews or in "cognitively induced" states [61–63]. Anxiety, stress, and conflict were associated with a decrease in skin temperature, while relaxation, security, and comfort were correlated with an increase. Thus it is difficult to know whether patients are learning skin temperature control or are simply learning a general relaxation response in which skin temperature change is merely a secondary consequence.

Awareness

In addition to the effects of relaxation, the contribution of other non-specific treatment factors such as "enhanced awareness" has become repeatedly apparent. In general, with extended practice in skin temperature control and relaxation, our patients became increasingly proficient in detecting the subtle internal indications of tension in day-to-day life. Such enhanced awareness provided the cues for initiating temperature/relaxation procedures, thereby short-circuiting the reaction. Catching tension levels in their embryonic stages thus contributed to overall stress reduction. The enhanced awareness also served as a sensitive barometer for recognizing environmental stressors (headache-triggering factors) and enabled the patients to cope more effectively through relaxation or avoidance of the stressful stimuli.

Increased awareness of internal states has been considered an essential step in the development of "cultivated low arousal" by Stoyva and Budzynski [64]. Furthermore, some authors have commented on the importance of facilitating internal awareness of rising tension states as part of learning to apply self-control techniques.

Cognitive set

The biofeedback paradigm should not be considered a simplistic mechanical technique involving the attachment of electrodes and automatic learning of physiological self-control, resulting in a subsequent cure of the problem. Rather, intertwined with the learning of physiological self-regulation lies a multilevel interaction of subject (patient), experimenter (therapist), and experimental situation (therapy) variables. All variables considered relevant in a typical therapeutic situation are in force in biofeedback, including subject expectations, faith in the doctor or treatment, motivation, suggestibility, therapist enthusiasm, instructions, credibility of the treatment rationale, and others.

These points have been illustrated by Taub [14], who reported a marked difference in the ability of a biofeedback therapist to successfully train subjects to warm their hands, depending on whether the therapist was impersonal and skeptical of the task or if she was warm, friendly, and confident about the feasibility of the task. Adler and Morrissey-Adler [65, 66], in particular, articulated the relationship between the biofeedback paradigm and psychotherapeutic variables.

Not least important among the complex therapeutic variables is the "cognitive set" of the patient. Migraine headache patients often turn to biofeedback after repeated failures in more traditional therapeutic modalities. There is a sense of fear and helplessness surrounding the headache attacks; the patients are victims without control over the situation; and, though hopeful, there is a background feeling that biofeedback will not succeed. Lazarus [45] addressed this often neglected issue of patient "cognitive appraisal" of the disease and therapy factors. Similarly Meichenbaum [44] stressed the role of cognitions and "self-statements" during biofeedback training. In the language of Meichenbaum, there tends to be a shift in cognitive self-statements from a sense of "learned helplessness" to "learned resourcefulness" following the patient's successful coping with migraine headaches. The patient develops a personal sense of self-control as one who takes an active role in modifying headache activity. These nonspecific effects on the patient cannot be underestimated in the overall treatment package.

Self-Report of Headache Data

One problem in assessing changes in headache activity is the necessity to rely on self-reported data. Patients' reports of headache frequency and analgesic consumption are probably more reliable and objective than self-reports of headache duration and especially pain intensity, which involve more judgmental factors. Perceived pain is influenced by many factors which have been reviewed elsewhere [67, 68]. However, the present data were based upon within-subject, pre- versus post-training comparisons in headache activity, and the biases in self-report data were assumed to remain constant for each subject over time. The relative change in headache activity was assessed by the experimenters rather than the patients and based upon headache rating charts filled out by the patients at the time of a headache or soon afterward [69].

Although in the majority of cases the patients' assessment of headache change was commensurate with the magnitude and pattern of change assessed by the experimenters, a minority of subjects were "poor witnesses" to the evolutionary nature of their headaches. The clearest examples of the dichotomy were illustrated by Subjects 3 and 10 in our study.

Subject 3 was trained to warm her hands but was pessimistic about outcome from the beginning. She was particularly alarmed about our institute's concern with "mental" sciences. During training, she consistently reported little change and was doubtful of success, though she persisted in training and home practice. When her headache scores were compiled, we found that despite her reports of "no change," her headache frequency had dropped 55 percent, there was a 50 percent decrease in the number of headache hours per month, with a nearly 20 percent decline in reported intensity. Interestingly, her consumption of ergotamine also dropped 50 percent, but she had increased analgesic consumption.

Subject 10 was extremely enthusiastic from the beginning of treatment and she had read about biofeedback. She was randomly placed in the hand-cooling group and during weekly debriefing sessions reported marked improvement. By the end of biofeedback training she reported that she had a marked reduction in headache activity and was thoroughly delighted with the results. Surprisingly, when the final data were tallied, frequency of her headaches was shown to have increased by 25 percent, there was a 23 percent increase in the number of headache hours per month, and each headache had increased in duration by an average of 30 percent compared to the pretraining baseline. However, her use of analgesics apparently reflected her beliefs because her consumption had declined by 95 percent.

The tendency for certain subjects to be poor evaluators of success points to the importance of the experimenters' assessing relative change over time in headache activity.

Absolute Versus Temperature Change

While the skin temperature factor is but one component in the therapeutic package, it has yet to be established whether the absolute degree of temperature attained or the change in skin temperature (delta-temperature) is the significant factor in behavioral methods of migraine management. In a majority of studies, the goal of the temperature training program was spontaneous hand-warming (delta-temperature) at the first indication of a migraine headache. However, data already reported in this chapter indicated only small and nonsignificant correlations between degree of temperature change and associated headache activity.

Conversely, many authorities agree that patients' ability to warm their hands in the 90° F range and above is a desirable skill. We are, however, aware of no published data that indicate a relationship between maintenance of a given absolute skin temperature and mitigation of migraine symptoms. Fahrion [70] uses combined training criteria, including the ability to maintain a skin temperature of at least 95.5° F for 10 minutes at a time and the ability to raise skin temperature at a rate of at least 1° F per minute. In our study, several individuals learned to abort potential headaches by warming their hands, and yet their absolute temperature generally remained in the 80° F range. The question of the relative importance of absolute versus delta-temperature has not been resolved. To answer the question would require constant sampling of hand temperature outside the laboratory setting during both headache and nonheadache periods.

Symptomatic Versus Prophylactic Application of Skin Temperature Control

Peripheral skin temperature control has both symptomatic and prophylactic applications to the management of migraine headache. In the present study, as in many others, patients typically are instructed to begin their hand-warming strategies at the earliest warning of an impending migraine attack and to practice hand-warming and relaxation daily whether or not they have had headaches.

The early reports by Sargent and associates [8] and others indicated that about 60 percent of migraine patients trained to warm their hands were able to abort their headache when they started hand-warming at the first indication of migraine attack. Turin and Johnson [28] reported the phenomenon of "chasing" a migraine with hand-warming. Similarly, in our study, 40 to 50 percent of the patients reported the ability to abort a migraine headache if they applied hand-warming during the headache aura or the initial phases of the headache. Only one person reported the ability to abort all such headaches reliably, while others could abort a percentage of their migraine headaches. Such an application is indicative of the symptomatic use of hand-warming.

It was also clear, however, that many migraineurs who failed in their attempts to abort headaches also experienced dramatically fewer headaches, and that the headaches were briefer and less intense. Thus it seems that daily practice of hand-warming and relaxation had a prophylactic effect. Additional evidence comes from an examination of aura activity in classic migraine patients and the initial phases of head pain in common migraine patients. If only symptomatic variables were at work, then patients would be expected to experience the same number of "beginnings" of headaches, even if the headaches were subsequently aborted. This was not the case, and many patients simply experienced fewer headaches independent of symptomatic applications. Improvement in migraine activity with consistent practice of hand-warming and relaxation was not unexpected. Data have been cited which indicate that the daily practice of a variety of traditional relaxation techniques alone may result in reduction of migraine headaches.

To conceptualize the effects of skin temperature control in terms of symptomatic and prophylactic effects has implications for both the theoretical mechanisms involved as well as clinical use of thermal biofeedback. It is interesting to speculate whether the symptomatic and prophylactic effects are mediated by different mechanisms. The prophylactic mechanism could be seen in terms of more efficient coping styles, recognition of stress-potentiating stimuli, and overall stress reduction, while the symptomatic mechanism of hand-warming might be mediated by an acute interruption of the biochemical events or cerebral hemodynamics known to occur in the initial stages of a migraine headache.

An intriguing speculation is that the skin temperature factor may play a differentially salient role in symptomatic and prophylactic applications. By way of indirect evidence, it is known that relaxation techniques alone may be effective in prophylactic reduction of migraine headache activity. However, we are not aware of any report of traditional relaxation techniques to abort a headache, while this symptomatic usage is generally reported with the hand-warming strategy. Such a concept may represent a consolidation of the relative roles of skin temperature control and relaxation in migraine management.

PHYSIOLOGICAL LEVEL OF ANALYSIS: REGIONAL CEREBRAL BLOOD FLOW

Is skin temperature self-regulation associated with change in regional cerebral blood flow?

Few studies have addressed the issue of mechanism with regard to the effects of hand-warming on migraine activity. Regardless of whether skin temperature or relaxation plays the dominant role in therapeutic gains, the question of physiological mechanism remains. To demonstrate a change in regional cerebral blood flow (rCBF) associated with skin temperature control may clarify the physiological basis of headache mitigation by skin temperature control.

In the migraine group, when mean hemispheric rCBF measures taken during the biofeedback run were compared to those of the relaxation/steady-state run, the left hemisphere of the hand-warming group exhibited a significant mean increase of 8.9 percent of gray matter flow while the right hemisphere increased a mean of 4.5 percent but did not reach statistical significance. An examination of the regional probe data indicated generalized increases of varying magnitudes, with significant increases in the left Sylvian-opercular and parietal areas.

These data indicate that there were indeed changes in cerebral blood flow associated with skin temperature control, although the significant changes were primarily in the left hemisphere. Changes in regional cerebral blood flow tend to support the theory that hand-warming strategies contribute to physiological changes in regional cerebral blood flow which may, in turn, be associated with an interruption of migraine headache activity.

The rCBF changes were small and subject to considerable variability, rendering interpretation of clinical significance difficult.

Hand-Warmers Versus Hand-Coolers

Do hand-warming and hand-cooling produce changes in rCBF which differ in magnitude, pattern, or direction?

This question addresses, on a physiological level, the issue of whether skin temperature is the most important variable in the behavioral treatment of migraine. Since hand-warmers and hand-coolers differed only in the direction of skin temperature control, they would presumably share all nonspecific treatment variables. If hand-warming is theoretically associated with a decrease in sympathetic nervous system outflow, and hand-cooling with an increase, then this difference would be reflected in rCBF. However, if both the hand-warming and hand-cooling groups shared a reduction in sympathetic outflow, then the two temperature groups would be expected to show similar rCBF changes.

The results indicated that the two groups of migraineurs did indeed differ in direction and magnitude of rCBF change. Figure 2 illustrates the pattern of rCBF change between the relaxation run and the biofeedback run for migraineurs trained to warm or cool their hands. In contrast to the significant 8.9 percent increase in the left hemisphere of the hand-warming group, the hand-coolers exhibited a negligible 1.4 percent increase. Right-hemisphere rCBF of the hand-warming group increased 4.5 percent while that of the cooling group decreased a mean 5.4 percent. In the hand-cooling group, neither hemispheric nor regional changes in rCBF reached significance, though patterns of increases and decreases differed from those of the hand-warming group.

The implication of these data is that hand-warming and hand-cooling

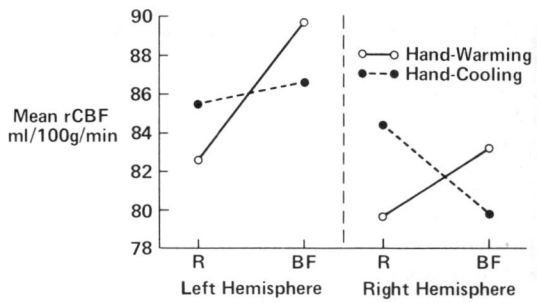

Figure 2. Mean hemispheric cerebral blood flow for relaxation (R) and biofeedback (BF) runs.

differ in terms of the associated magnitude, pattern, and direction of rCBF changes, which suggests that the skin temperature factor (or its influence on relaxation) may have a significant role in treatment of migraine.

rCBF Patterns in Normal Versus Migraine Patients

The original study on the relationship between peripheral skin temperature control and rCBF was carried out with normal subjects [15] and subsequently repeated with migraineurs [16]. The use of an identical paradigm in both studies allowed for a direct comparison of these groups. In contrast to the rCBF changes of the migraine groups, the normal groups were found to differ markedly in magnitude and pattern of rCBF changes associated with skin temperature self-regulation.

In the normal group, neither the subjects trained to warm or to cool their hands demonstrated a consistent change in left hemisphere rCBF (warmers, 0.4 percent; coolers, −2.9 percent). In contrast, the right hemispheres of both temperature groups showed consistent decreases of similar magnitude (warmers, −4.8 percent; coolers, −4.0 percent). On a probe-by-probe basis, the left and right hemispheres of the two temperature groups presented a mixed picture of increases and decreases.

Thus, in the normal groups studied, hand-warmers and hand-coolers tended to demonstrate similar hemispheric patterns of change, especially in the right hemisphere. These data in normals suggested that the skin temperature factor did not differentially affect rCBF. These patterns were not borne out in migraineurs, who did show a difference between hand-warmers and hand-coolers. In both studies, negligible fluctuations in mean arterial blood pressure and partial pressure of carbon dioxide could not account for the rCBF changes.

Indirect evidence in the literature indicates that normal subjects differ from migraineurs in terms of vasomotor reactivity. Early research by Tunis and Wolff [71] documented differences between migraineurs (during headache-free intervals) and normal subjects in terms of pulse amplitude lability of the temporal arteries. While differing widely in methods, several studies reviewed by Dalessio [4] and Bakal [72] reveal that migraineurs exhibit abnormalities in vascular reflex vasodilation and vasoconstriction in response to the application of hot and cold thermal stimuli respectively [73-76]. The implication of this research was that, compared to normals, migraineurs manifest a general deficit or instability in peripheral vasomotor control [2], a condition thought to be critical in the pathophysiology of migraine headache [4]. However, the conclusions of these studies have been challenged on methodological grounds by Morley and Phil [77], while in other studies conducted with similar paradigms no differences were found between normal subjects and migraineurs [78, 79]. More recently, Price and Tursky [80], studying skin temperature feedback, found a marked difference between normals and migraine patients in both digital and temporal artery blood volume changes. Similarly, other researchers have found migraine patients to show a more stereotypic physiological response pattern to various tasks [81] and differences in classical conditioning ability of digital pulse volume [82] in comparison to normal controls.

Relationship between Skin Temperature and rCBF

During the ten-minute measurement period of rCBF, peripheral skin temperature change scores were calculated by subtracting the absolute skin temperature at minute 1 from that at minute 10. Data from both normal and migraine studies indicate that the temperature groups successfully manipulated their skin temperature during biofeedback runs. In contrast, during the relaxation runs there tended to be little change in skin temperature for all groups, as expected.

In the normal group, the peak warming trends during rCBF measurements ranged from $0.7°$ to $3.7°$ C and the cooling group decreased their skin temperature a peak of $-0.1°$ to $-1.9°$ C. In the migraine group, the hand warmers increased their skin temperature a peak of $0°$ to $3.0°$ C while the peak cooling trends for the hand-cooling group ranged from $-0.2°$ to $-0.8°$ C. In both studies, the two temperature groups were able to change their skin temperatures in significantly opposite directions, despite the moderately tense conditions and unfamiliar environment of the blood flow laboratory.

Is there a correlation between the magnitude of skin temperature changes during the biofeedback run and associated change in rCBF?

The correlational data indicated an additional difference between normals and migraineurs. In the normal group, the change in skin temperature correlated 0.59 ($p < 0.1$) with left hemisphere mean blood flow and -0.36 (n.s.) with right hemisphere change. The correlations between skin temperature and rCBF for the migraine group are illustrated in Table 2. Though modest, the greater relationship appeared between the magnitude of skin temperature change and right hemisphere blood flow, which is not surprising as the right hemisphere rCBF tended to show an increase for hand-warmers and a decrease for hand-coolers.

Relationship between Headache Variables and Change in rCFB

Table 3 illustrates the correlations between changes in mean hemispheric rCBF during skin temperature self-regulation and the mean percentage of improvement of each headache variable. These data have meaning if one assumes that the observed rCBF changes are reliable across attempts to change skin temperature.

The left hemispheric change in mean rCBF correlated highest with the two headache duration indices and one headache intensity index, while change in the right hemisphere correlated highest with an intensity

Table 2

Correlations between Regional Cerebral Blood Flow and Skin Temperature Self-Regulation during CBF Run

Probes	Skin Temperature Change	
	Left Hemisphere	Right Hemisphere
Frontal	.11	.50
Precentral	−.49	.14
Parietal	.32	.67 ($p < .05$)
Sylvian-Opercular	−.03	.33
Posterior Temporal	.52 ($p < .1$)	.29
Occipital	.47	.38
Inferior Temporal	.03	.52 ($p < .1$)
Brainstem/Cerebellar	−.06	−.08
Mean Hemispheric Flow	.27	.58 ($p < .1$)

Table 3

Correlations between Hemispheric Cerebral Blood Flow and Headache Variables

	Analgesic Units per Month	Mean Analgesic Units per Headache	Frequency per Month	Headache Hours per Month	Mean Hours per Headache	Intensity Hours per Month	Mean Intensity Hours per Headache
Left Hemisphere CBF	−.31	−.12	−.18	−.53 ($p < .1$)	−.78 ($p < .01$)	−.61 ($p < .05$)	−.31
Right Hemisphere CBF	−.09	−.11	−.13	−.36	−.36	−.39	−.65 ($p < .05$)

index as well. All the correlations were negative, indicating that increases in hemispheric rCBF were associated with a decline in the headache variable.

Relationship between Hand Training and rCBF

It has been pointed out that, in the migraine group, the largest and most consistent changes in rCBF occurred in the left hemisphere during hand-warming. The left hemisphere is contralateral to the hand trained in skin temperature control. One possible interpretation is that the left hemisphere change may simply reflect an increase in metabolic demands of the left hemisphere gray matter in association with selective attention to the right hand. This does not seem to be a viable hypothesis. Normal subjects who were exposed to the identical training paradigm and who also warmed their hands successfully did not show an augmented increase in left hemisphere flow. In addition, the cooling groups in both studies were also trained on their right hand, yet they did not show notable left hemisphere increases. There was also no correlation between skin temperature and left hemisphere rCBF change illustrated in Table 2. In future research it would be worthwhile to train skin temperature on the left hand and look for reversals in hemispheric patterns.

Implications for Mechanism

Hemodynamics in migraine headache

The theoretical mechanisms to account for reduction in migraine headache activity after acute application of hand-warming strategies are unclear at best. They are based in part on the known alterations in intracerebral and extracerebral hemodynamics which occur before, during, and after a migraine episode.

Evidence reviewed thus far has suggested that migraineurs have an exaggerated vascular responsiveness and variability, which may reflect a general instability of the autonomic nervous system.

Research by Tunis and Wolff [71] has indicated that the temporal artery branches of the external carotid system tend to show increased instability 36 to 74 hours prior to onset of a migraine headache, which turns into a fluctuating pattern of alternating vasoconstriction and vasodilatation about six hours before the headache attack.

Quantitative measures of cerebral vascular hemodynamics during a migraine episode tend to support Wolff's vascular theory of migraine [4]. During the prodromal phase of a classic migraine, significant reductions in CBF have been verified by the ^{133}Xe intracarotid injection method [85–89] and by the noninvasive ^{133}Xe inhalation technique [90, 91]. During the headache phase, compensatory vasodilatation and hyperfusion have been documented in both extracranial artery distribution [4, 71, 92] and in intracranial circulation via the ^{133}Xe injection method [85, 88, 89], as well as the ^{133}Xe inhalation method [91, 93]. Recent evidence presented by Sakai and Meyer [93], using serial measurements of CBF, showed that intracerebral blood flow may remain significantly increased for up to 48 hours after the headache subsides (see chapter 1, this volume).

Hypothesized mechanisms of thermal biofeedback

Although they differ on exact mechanism, theoreticians seem to agree that volitional increase of skin temperature of the hands reflects a reduction of sympathetic nervous system outflow. Stress and associated sympathetic nervous system activity has been implicated in the pathogenesis of migraine headache.

Sargent and co-workers [8] were among the earliest to posit that hand-warming involved a generalized reduction of excessive sympathetic outflow, which included a "normalization of homeostatic balance in hypothalamic control centers." Given neuroanatomic and physiologic evidence that the peripheral vascular structures are innervated primarily by the sympathetic nervous system [94], and that the effect of increased sympathetic activation results in peripheral vasoconstriction, evidence suggested that the hands could only be voluntarily warmed in association with a decline of sympathetic outflow (mediated by the hypothalamus), which allows the peripheral blood vessels to dilate. Presumably, the effect generalizes to the cephalic vascular system as well and produces a physiological state incompatible with the neurochemical and/or hemodynamic chain of events in migraine headache.

Recent research by Sovak et al. and Dalessio et al. [95, 96] has provided further evidence that hand-warming is associated with a general decrease in tonic sympathetic outflow. These authors measured heart rate patterns and vascular reactivity of skin and muscle during hand-warming. Fahrion [97] suggested that a general relaxation of sympathetic outflow results in a decline in headache activity through the stabilizing effect on the vasomotor tone of the cranial arteries. Such a mechanism may explain the symptomatic aborting of a headache and prevention of future episodes of headache through regular practice.

Other authors have focused on the more symptomatic applications of hand-warming and have hypothesized an associated vasoconstriction or vasodilation of the cranial arteries, depending upon the stage of headache. Stroebel and Glueck [98], for example, proposed that volitional warming of the hands prevents the excessive degree of intracerebral vasoconstriction in the prodromal stage, preventing the release of neurokinins and related neuroactive substances which would result in the reactive vasodilatation associated with the headache phase.

Mechanism suggested by the present study

Our results with migraine patients indicated that hand-warming was associated with bilateral increases in cerebral blood flow, with greater increases occurring in the left hemisphere. These data are compatible with Stroebel and Glueck's hypothesis [98]. Bilateral hemispheric vasodilatation associated with hand-warming may serve to interrupt, reverse, or produce a state incompatible with the intracerebral vasoconstriction characteristic of the pre-headache stage.

A number of questions remain unanswered. For example, it is unknown whether the increase in CBF observed with hand-warming is mediated by active vasodilation or inhibition of vasoconstriction. Nor is it known if the effects on rCBF are mediated by direct neurogenic interventions or indirectly through changes in the neurochemical milieu. It is clear, however, that the mechanism is complex, given the bilateral hemisphere changes of unequal magnitude and direction as well as the pattern of regional changes.

It is unlikely that the simple vasodilation of peripheral vascular structures should influence the powerful autoregulatory mechanisms governing CBF. More plausible explanations should be couched in terms of the complex interactions among neurogenic, biochemical, neural metabolism, and myogenic influences [25]. The exact contribution of these factors and their interactions in the regulation of CBF is unclear. Neurogenic influences would imply direct changes in the vessels due to shifts in sympathetic nervous outflow. Metabolic influences may result from increased regional metabolism in association with mental strategies used in hand-warming. Biochemical influences may be mediated by associated changes in circulating catecholamines.

Recent evidence on the biochemistry of biofeedback supports a biochemical rationale for the influence of relaxation on migraine activity (see chapter 8, this volume). Changes in serotonin, norepinephrine, epinephrine, histamine, prostaglandins, neurokinins, etc. have been implicated in the development of migraine. A change in the biochemical milieu mediated by hand-warming could conceivably interrupt the chain of biochemical events at any point.

Headache Stage and Site of Therapeutic Action

A key issue is whether hand-warming primarily affects the intracranial or extracranial vasculature in the symptomatic treatment of migraine. Stroebel and Glueck [98] suggest that the effects occur on intracranial vessels in the prodromal stage of a headache. Similarly, the studies of CBF and biofeedback have been directed toward intracerebral blood flow changes. Corresponding extracranial effects on the scalp surface were not measured.

A related issue is the question whether hand-warming is specific to stage of headache. Given the vast difference in hemodynamics and biochemistry between the prodromal and headache stages of a migraine attack, to specify whether the success of hand-warming is limited to the prodromal stage (characterized by intracerebral vasoconstriction) or remains effective during the early headache phase (characterized by both intra- and extracerebral vasodilation) has implications for understanding the theoretical mechanisms and the vascular system involved. Sargent et al. [8] reported that, once headache pain has begun, it is difficult to abort the headache. Stroebel and Glueck [98] believe that biofeedback may help to reduce activation level or reactive muscular bracing against pain. Headache pain is believed to serve as a distraction, circumventing successful self-regulation. In our study, however, the hand-warming ability of one subject was measured during a migraine headache. Despite pain, she was able to warm her hands 3.0° C with no effect on the head pain, but in fact produced a worsened throbbing because of intense concentration. Two subjects who had common migraine reported that they succeeded in aborting their headache after the pain had begun. This occurred only when hand-warming was done immediately at onset of pain and if the pain had begun slowly.

Biofeedback for Hand-Warming Versus Cephalic Vasoconstriction

Hand-warming is believed to reflect a generalized decline in sympathetic nervous system outflow which may, in turn, influence the tone of the intracerebral artery system. An alternative technique, learned vasoconstriction of the extracranial vasculature (i.e., decrease in blood pulse volume of the temporal arteries), seems to be a specific technique directed toward another vascular system and a different headache phase.

The rationale is based on the observation that headache pain is associated with vasodilation of the superficial scalp arteries and that learned vasoconstriction of these arteries may reduce headache intensity. Feuerstein and Adams [99] proposed that the mechanism may involve increased vascular tone, reducing lability and reactivity of the cephalic vasomotor system to environmental stressors.

Early research with normal volunteers [100] and migraineurs [101] (in asymptomatic state) indicated that learned modification of the superficial temporal artery pulse volume is possible. Though differing widely in measurement techniques and training paradigms, several recent studies [99–105] indicated that migraineurs trained in extracranial "vasoconstriction" may experience significant improvement in headache activity. The data seem promising, but larger studies are required with control groups and follow-up. Data on headache stage relationships are also lacking. As is true for hand-warming, learned "vasoconstriction" of the extracranial arteries has not been proved superior to relaxation.

While hand-warming and learned reductions in extracranial artery pulse volume seem to involve different mechanisms, recent evidence [95, 96] indicates that there may be more overlap in the two techniques than was suspected. Using a combination of Doppler ultrasound techniques and photoplethysmography, patterns of vascular behavior were measured in the supraorbital and superficial temporal arteries in the scalp, radial and brachial arteries in the arms, and digital arterial beds. When migraineurs trained in hand-warming attempted to raise their peripheral skin temperature, associated vasodilatation was found in the digits and vasoconstriction in the scalp arteries in patients who improved clinically. This pattern was labeled the "adaptation-relaxation reflex" and was considered to represent a retraining of the autonomic nervous system to produce a decrease in sympathetic tone. In patients who did not improve, a vasodilatation pattern was elicited in both scalp and digits in association with hand-warming. Such evidence seems to unite the hand-warming and cephalic vasomotor constriction paradigms, since the evidence by Sovak et al. [95] implicates the occurrence of both processes during hand-warming in clinically improved migraineurs.

CONCLUSIONS

Two groups of migraineurs and normal volunteers were randomly divided into hand-warming and hand-cooling groups and given extensive biofeedback training. Each subject was then given a baseline regional cerebral blood flow measurement while relaxing and a second one while self-regulating skin temperature in the trained direction. Issues of mechanism and significance of the skin temperature factor were explored together with additional tangential issues. Normal volunteers were compared to migraineurs and hand-warmers to hand-coolers on two levels of analysis: behavioral (headache: pre- versus post-training comparisons) and physiological (rCBF: rest versus biofeedback runs).

Conclusions and speculations from the study are:

Behavioral Level of Analysis

1. Though trained to alter their skin temperature in opposite directions, the migraineurs in both hand-warming and hand-cooling groups experienced substantial improvement in medication consumed, headache duration, and one index of headache intensity. As for headache frequency and another index of intensity, hand-warmers tended to improve and hand-coolers tended to worsen. There was considerable variation in individual patterns of headache symptom change.

2. Improvement in headache activity was ascribed largely to nonspecific treatment effects and, to a lesser extent, temperature-specific effects. We speculated that relaxation, increased awareness, and shifts in cognitive set were the major active components of the nonspecific treatment effects. The magnitude of the learned skin temperature changes bore little relationship to the amount of headache improvement. The relative importance to migraine activity of absolute skin temperature versus learned change in skin temperature remains unclear. The exact significance of the skin temperature factor must await studies involving constant in vivo sampling of skin temperature during headache-free and headache periods.

3. Hand-warming has both symptomatic and prophylactic applications to the management of migraine, and it is possible that they involve

different mechanisms of action. It was further speculated that the relative importance of a skin temperature factor may differ between symptomatic and prophylactic applications.

Physiological Level of Analysis

4. Relative to relaxation runs, changes in regional cerebral blood flow were associated with attempts to self-regulate skin temperature. Differences were found between hand-warmers and hand-coolers in the magnitude and direction of rCBF change. There was a slight correlation between change in skin temperature and rCBF change.

5. Though exposed to identical paradigms, normal subjects and migraineurs displayed different patterns of rCBF change in association with skin temperature control.

6. Relationships were found between certain headache variables and changes in rCBF.

7. These data support an earlier hypothesis that warming the hands may serve to prevent the extreme degree of intracerebral vasoconstriction, thereby circumventing the reactive vasodilatation associated with the headache phase. These changes were believed to be mediated by alterations in sympathetic outflow.

Our conclusions should be considered conservatively because the number of normal and migraine subjects was limited and thus the study requires replication with larger groups. Considerable variability was found in the magnitude of skin temperature changes, patterns of headache activity, and patterns of regional cerebral blood flow.

REFERENCES

1. Ad Hoc Committee on Classification of Headache. *JAMA* 179:717–718, 1962.
2. Selby G, Lance JW: Observations of 500 cases of migraine and allied vascular headache. *J Neurol Neurosurg Psychiatry* 23:23–32, 1960.
3. Lance JW, Anthony M: Some clinical aspects of migraine: A prospective survey of 500 patients. *Arch Neurol* 15:356–361, 1966.
4. Dalessio DJ: *Wolff's Headache and Other Head Pain*, 3rd Ed. New York, Oxford Press, 1972.
5. Ray WJ, Raczynski JM, Rogers T, Kimball WH: *Evaluation of Clinical Biofeedback*. New York, Plenum Press, 1979.
6. Sargent JD, Green EE, Walters ED: The use of autogenic feedback training in a pilot study of migraine and tension headaches. *Headache* 12:120–125, 1972.
7. Sargent JD, Green EE, Walters ED: Preliminary report on the use of autogenic

feedback training in the treatment of migraine and tension headaches. *Psychosom Med* 35:129–135, 1973.
8. Sargent JD, Walters ED, Green EE: Psychosomatic self-regulation of migraine headaches. *Seminars in Psychiatry* 5:415–427, 1973.
9. Price KP: Biofeedback and migraine, in Gatchel RJ, Price KP (eds): *Clinical Applications of Biofeedback: Appraisal and Status.* New York, Pergamon Press, 1979.
10. Diamond S, Diamond-Falk J, DeVeno T: Biofeedback in the treatment of vascular headache. *Biofeedback Self Regul* 3:385–408, 1978.
11. Board of Directors, American Association for the Study of Headache: Biofeedback therapy. *Headache* 18:107, 1978.
12. Blanchard EG, Young LD: Clinical applications of biofeedback training: A review of evidence. *Arch Gen Psychiatry* 30:574–589, 1974.
13. Miller NE: Biofeedback and visceral learning. *Annu Rev Psychol* 29:373–404, 1978.
14. Taub E: Self regulation of human tissue temperature, in Schwartz GE, Beatty J (eds): *Biofeedback: Theory and Research.* New York, Academic Press, 1977.
15. Largen JW, Mathew RJ, Dobbins K, Meyer JS, Claghorn JL: Skin temperature self-regulation and non-invasive regional cerebral blood flow. *Headache* 18:203–210, 1978.
16. Mathew RJ, Largen JW, Dobbins K, Meyer JS, Sakai F, Claghorn JL: Biofeedback control of skin temperature and cerebral blood flow in migraine. *Headache* 20:19–28, 1980.
17. Largen JW, Mathew RJ, Dobbins K, Claghorn JL: Specific and non-specific effects of skin temperature control in migraine management. *Headache* 21:36–44, 1981.
18. Bakal DA, Kaganov JA: Muscle contraction and migraine headache: Psychophysiological comparison. *Headache* 17:208–215, 1977.
19. Budzynski TH, Stoyva JM, Adler CS, Mullaney DJ: EMG biofeedback and tension headache: A controlled outcome study. *Seminars in Psychiatry* 5:397–409, 1973.
20. Jacobson E: *Progressive Relaxation.* Chicago, University of Chicago Press, 1938.
21. Obrist WD, Thompson HK, King CH, Wang HS: Determination of regional cerebral blood flow by inhalation of ^{133}Xenon. *Circ Res* 20:124–135, 1967.
22. Obrist WD, Thompson HK, Wang HS, Wilkinson WE: Regional cerebral blood flow by ^{133}Xenon inhalation. *Stroke* 6:245–256, 1975.
23. Meyer JS, Ishihara N, Deshmukh VD, Naritomi H, Sakai F, Hsu M-C, Pollack P: Improved method for noninvasive measurement of regional cerebral blood flow by ^{133}Xenon inhalation (Part 1). *Stroke* 9:205–210, 1978.
24. Meyer JS: Improved method for noninvasive measurement of regional cerebral blood flow by ^{133}Xenon inhalation (Part 2). *Stroke* 9:205–210, 1978.
25. Deshmukh VD, Meyer JS: *Noninvasive Measurement of Regional Cerebral Blood Flow in Man.* New York, Spectrum, 1978.

26. Wickramasekera IE: Temperature feedback for the control of migraine. *Journal of Behavior Therapy and Experimental Psychiatry* 4:343–345, 1973.
27. Diamond S, Medina JL: The treatment of headache with different modalities of biofeedback therapy (abstract). *Headache* 16:80–81, 1976.
28. Turin A, Johnson WG: Biofeedback therapy for migraine headache. *Arch Gen Psychiatry* 33:517–519, 1976.
29. Andreychuk T, Skriver C: Hypnosis and biofeedback in the treatment of migraine headache. *Int J Clin Exp Hypn* 23:172–183, 1975.
30. Mullinix JM, Norton BJ, Hack S, Fishman MA: Skin temperature biofeedback and migraine. *Headache* 17:242–244, 1978.
31. Werbach MR, Sandweiss JH: Peripheral temperature of migraineurs undergoing relaxation training. *Headache* 18:211–214, 1978.
32. Blanchard EB, Theobald DE, Williamson DA, Silver BV, Brown DA: Temperature biofeedback in the treatment of migraine headaches. *Arch Gen Psychiatry* 35:581–588, 1978.
33. Silver BV, Blanchard EB, Williamson DA, Theobald DE, Brown DA: Temperature biofeedback and relaxation training in the treatment of migraine headaches: One year follow-up. *Biofeedback Self Regul* 4:359–366, 1979.
34. Coyne L, Sargent JD, Sergerson J, Obourn R: Relative potency scale for analgesic drugs: Use of psychophysiological procedure with clinical judgements. *Headache* 16:70–71, 1976.
35. Lacey JI, Bateman DE, VanLehn R: Autonomic response specificity: An experimental study. *Psychosom Med* 15:8–21, 1973.
36. Kewman DG, Roberts AH: Skin temperature biofeedback and migraine headaches: A double-blind study. Presented to Biofeedback Society of America Annual Meeting, 1979.
37. Silver BV, Blanchard EB: Biofeedback and relaxation treatment of psychophysiological disorders: Or are the machines really necessary? *Journal of Behavioral Medicine* 1:217–239, 1978.
38. Budzynski TH: Biofeedback strategies in headache treatment, in Basmajian JV (ed): *Biofeedback—Principles and Practice for Clinicians*. Baltimore, Williams & Wilkins, 1979.
39. Friedman AP: Headache, in Baker AB, Baker LH (eds): *Clinical Neurology*. New York, Harper & Row, 1976.
40. Shapiro AK: Placebo effects in medicine, psychotherapy, psychoanalysis, in Bergin AE, Garfield SL (eds): *Handbook of Psychotherapy and Behavior Change*. New York, Wiley, 1971.
41. Wickramasekera IE: Biofeedback, behavior therapy and hypnosis: Convergences and the placebo response, in Wickramasekera IE (ed): *Biofeedback, Behavior Therapy and Hypnosis: Potentiating the Verbal Control of Behavior for Clinicians*. Chicago, Nelson-Hall, 1976.
42. Maletzky BM: Behavior recording as treatment: A brief note. *Behavior Therapy* 5:107–111, 1974.
43. Zimmerman J, Levitt AE: Why not give your client a counter: A survey of what happened when we did. *Behav Res Ther* 13:333–337, 1975.

44. Meichenbaum D: Cognitive factors in biofeedback therapy. *Biofeedback Self Regul* 1:201–216, 1976.
45. Lazarus RS: A cognitively oriented psychologist looks at biofeedback. *Self Regul* 1:201–216, 1976.
46. Adler CS, Adler SM: Biofeedback-psychotherapy for the treatment of headaches: A 5-year follow-up. *Headache* 16:189–191, 1976.
47. Diamond S, Diamond-Falk J, DeVeno T: The value of biofeedback in the treatment of chronic headache: A five-year retrospective study. *Headache* 19:90–96, 1979.
48. Solbach P, Sargent JD: A follow-up evaluation of the Menninger pilot migraine study using thermal training. *Headache* 17:198–202, 1977.
49. Lance JW, Anthony M, Somerville B: Thermographic, hormonal, and clinical studies in migraine. *Headache* 10:93–104, 1970.
50. Mitchell KR, White RJ: Behavioral self-management: An application to the problem of migraine headache. *Behavior Therapy* 8:213–221, 1977.
51. Benson H, Beary JF, Carol MP: The relaxation response. *Psychiatry* 37:37–46, 1974.
52. Woolfolk, RL: Psychophysiological correlates of meditation. *Arch Gen Psychiatry* 32:1326–1333, 1975.
53. Luthe W: Autogenic training: Method, research and application in medicine. *Am J Psychiatry* 17:174–195, 1963.
54. Benson H, Malvea BP, Graham JR: Physiologic correlates of meditation and their clinical effects in headache: An ongoing investigation. *Headache* 13:23–24, 1973.
55. Hay KM, Madders J: Migraine treated by relaxation therapy. *J R Coll Gen Pract* 21:664–669, 1971.
56. Warner G, Lance JW: Relaxation therapy in migraine and chronic tension headache. *Med J Aust* 1:298–301, 1975.
57. Lutker ER: Treatment of migraine headache by conditioned relaxation: A case study. *Behavior Therapy* 2:592–593, 1971.
58. Tarler-Benlolo L: The role of relaxation in biofeedback training: A critical review of the literature. *Psychol Bull* 85:727–755, 1978.
59. Keefe FJ: Biofeedback versus instructional control of skin temperature. *J Behav Med* 1:383–390, 1978.
60. Surwit RS, Pilon RN, Fenton CH: Behavioral treatment of Raynaud's disease. *J Behav Med* 1:323–335, 1978.
61. Mittelman B, Wolff HG: Affective states and skin temperature: Experimental study of subjects with "cold hands" and Raynaud's syndrome. *Psychosom Med* 1:271–292, 1939.
62. Pinsker EJ, Russell HL: The effect of positive verbal strokes on finger tip skin temperature: Objective measurement of interpersonal interaction. *Transactional Analysis J* 8:306–309, 1978.
63. Crawford DG, Friesen DD, Tomlinson-Keasey C: Effects of cognitively induced anxiety on hand temperature. *Biofeedback and Self Regul* 2:139–146, 1977.
64. Stoyva J, Budzynski T: Cultivated low arousal—an antistress response?, in DiCara,

LV (ed): *Recent Advances in Limbic and Autonomic Nervous System Research.* New York, Plenum Press, 1974.
65. Adler CS, Morrissey-Adler S: Strategies in general psychiatry, in Basmajian JV (ed): *Biofeedback—Principles and Practice for Clinicians.* Baltimore, Williams & Wilkins, 1979.
66. Adler CS, Morrissey-Adler S: Biofeedback and psychosomatic disorders, in Basmajian JV (ed): *Biofeedback—Principles and Practice for Clinicians.* Baltimore, Williams & Wilkins, 1979.
67. Weisenberg M: Pain and pain control. *Psychol Bull* 84:1004–1008, 1977.
68. Bonica JS: *Pain.* Research Publications: Association for Research in Nervous and Mental Disease, vol. 58. New York, Raven Press, 1980.
69. Andrasik F, Holroyd KA: Reliability and concurrent validity of headache questionnaire data. *Headache* 20:44–46, 1980.
70. Fahrion SL: Autogenic biofeedback treatment for migraine. *Mayo Clin Proc* 52:776–784, 1977.
71. Tunis MM, Wolff HG: Studies on headache: Long term observations of the reactivity of the cranial arteries in subjects with vascular headache of the migraine type. *Arch Neurol Psychiatry* 70:551–557, 1953.
72. Bakal DA: Headache: A biopsychological perspective. *Psychol Bull* 82:369–382, 1975.
73. Appenzeller O, Davidson K, Marshall J: Reflex vasomotor abnormalities in the hands of migrainous subjects. *J Neurol Neurosurg Psychiatry* 26:447–450, 1963.
74. Appenzeller O: Vasomotor function in migraine. *Headache* 9:155–157, 1969.
75. Downey JA, Frewin DB: Vascular responses in the hands of patients suffering from migraine. *J Neurol Neurosurg Psychiatry* 38:258–263, 1972.
76. Elliot K, Frewin DB, Downey JA: Reflex vasomotor responses in the hands of patients suffering from migraine. *Headache* 13:188–196, 1974.
77. Morley S, Phil M: Migraine: A generalized vasomotor dysfunction? *Headache* 17:71–74, 1977.
78. French EB, Lassers BW, Desia MG: Vasomotor responses in the hand of migraine subjects. *J Neurol Neurosurg Psychiatry* 30:276–278, 1967.
79. Hockaday JM, MacMilliam AL, Whitty CWM: Vasomotor reflex in idiopathic and hormone dependent migraine. *Lancet* 1:1023–1026, 1967.
80. Price RP, Tursky B: Vascular reactivity of migraineurs and nonmigraineurs: A comparison of responses to self control procedures. *Headache* 16:210–217, 1976.
81. Cohen MJ, Rickles WH, McArthur DL: Evidence for physiological response stereotype in migraine headache. *Psychosom Med* 40:344–354, 1978.
82. Price KP, Clarke LK: Classical conditioning of digital pulse volume in migraineurs and normal controls. *Headache* 19:328–332, 1979.
83. Edmeads J: Cerebral blood flow in migraine. *Headache* 17:148–152, 1977.
84. Kudrow L: Current aspects of migraine headache. *Psychosomatics* 19:48–57, 1978.
85. Skinhøj E: Hemodynamic studies within the brain during migraine. *Arch Neurol* 29:95–98, 1973.

86. Simard D, Paulson OB: Cerebral vasomotor paralysis during migraine attack. Arch Neurol 29:207–209, 1973.
87. Norris JW, Hackinski BC, Cooper PW: Changes in cerebral blood flow during a migraine attack. Br Med J 3:676–684, 1975.
88. Mathew NT, Hrastnik F, Meyer JS: Regional cerebral blood flow in the diagnosis of vascular headache. Headache 15:252–260, 1976.
89. Edmeads J: Cerebral blood flow in migraine. Headache 17:148–152, 1977.
90. O'Brien MD: The relationship between aura blood flow changes in the prodrome of migraine. Headache 11:90–91, 1971.
91. O'Brien MD: Cerebral blood flow changes in migraine. Headache 10:139–143, 1971.
92. Elkind AH, Friedman AP, Grossman J: Cutaneous blood flow in vascular headaches of the migraine type. Neurology 14:24–30, 1964.
93. Sakai F, Meyer JS: Regional cerebral hemodynamics during migraine and cluster headaches measured by the ^{133}Xe inhalation method. Headache 18:122–132, 1978.
94. Greenfield AD: The circulation through the skin, in Handbook of Physiology. Washington, American Physiological Society, 1963.
95. Sovak M, Kunzel M, Sternbach RA, Dalessio DJ: Is volitional manipulation of hemodynamics a valid rationale for biofeedback therapy of migraine? Headache 18:197–202, 1978.
96. Dalessio DJ, Kunzel M, Sternbach RA, Sovak M: Conditioned adaptation, relaxation, reflex and migraine therapy. JAMA 242:2102–2104, 1979.
97. Fahrion SL: Autogenic biofeedback for migraine. Psychiatric Annals 8:219–234, 1978.
98. Stroebel CF, Glueck BC: Psychophysiological rationale for the application of biofeedback in the alleviation of pain, in Weisenberg M, Tursky B (eds): Pain: New Perspectives in Therapy and Research, New York, Plenum, 1976.
99. Feuerstein M, Adams HE: Cephalic vasomotor feedback in the modification of migraine headache. Biofeedback and Self-Regulation 2:241–254, 1977.
100. Christie DJ, Kotses H: Bidirectional operant conditioning of the cephalic vasomotor response. J Psychosom Res 17:167–170, 1973.
101. Koppman JW, McDonald RD, Kunzel MG: Voluntary regulation of temporal artery diameter by migraine patients. Headache 14:133–138, 1974.
102. Friar LR, Beatty J: Migraine: Management by trained control of vasoconstriction. J Consult Clin Psychol 44:46–53, 1976.
103. Feuerstein M, Adams HE, Beiman I: Cephalic vasomotor and electromyographic feedback in the treatment of combined muscle contraction and migraine headaches in a geriatric case. Headache 16:232–237, 1976.
104. Sturgis ET, Tollison CD, Adams HC: Modification of combined migraine muscle contraction headache using BVP and EMG feedback. J Appl Beh Analysis 11:215–223, 1978.
105. Bilo R, Adams HE: Modification of migraine headaches by cephalic blood volume pulse and EMG biofeedback. J Consult Clin Psychol 48:51–57, 1980.

… Copyright © 1981, Spectrum Publications, Inc.
Treatment of Migraine

Chapter 8
Biochemistry of Biofeedback Treatment

ROY J. MATHEW, M.D.
BENG T. HO, PH.D.

Biofeedback came to be widely accepted as an effective form of treatment for migraine headaches after the initial report of its antimigraine action was substantiated by several other groups [1, 2, 3, 4]. Biofeedback clinics have sprung up all over the country, and most headache clinics now offer biofeedback treatment. While the clinician uses skin-temperature biofeedback with confidence in its efficacy, the researcher remains doubtful. The application of skin-temperature biofeedback in treating migraine headache raises several issues that need theoretical clarification.

Volitional control over autonomic functions forms the basis for biofeedback therapy. Since all human beings possess a certain degree of conscious control over such involuntary functions as skin temperature by changes in skeletomuscular tone, the additional degree of control gained through biofeedback training is difficult to evaluate. Long before biofeedback came into being, it was known that relaxation techniques such as transcendental meditation were capable of inducing changes in autonomic functions [5–7]. Relaxation is an important aspect of biofeedback training. The question is whether or not biofeedback can give volitional control over a physiological function such as skin temperature, over and above the effect of relaxation.

In earlier animal studies, the influence of the skeletomuscular system on the autonomic nervous system was circumvented by paralyzing the muscles with curare; for obvious reasons this cannot be done in human beings [8]. Thus, contamination by the nonautonomic skeletomuscular system is the main stumbling block in examining the possibility of autonomic nervous system training in human beings. The task is rendered even more intricate by other elements. Autonomic functions such as skin temperature are influenced by several nonspecific factors such as ambient temperature and humidity, metabolic rate, body temperature, exercise, tobacco use, and endogenous biological rhythms. Consequently, these functions fluctuate spontaneously by wide margins from moment to moment.

Available evidence certainly does not warrant the conclusion that biofeedback training gives absolute and total control over previously involuntary functions. The issue in question is one of increase in the degree of control following biofeedback training. Demonstrations of degrees of control over a function which fluctuates widely and frequently and is influenced by several nonspecific factors is difficult to quantify unless the degree of control is very high and consistent. There is no literature on the important issue of the length of time over which volitional induced changes in the autonomic function can be maintained. It is questionable whether an evanescent shift in skin temperature, for example, will be sufficient to reverse vasomotor pathology such as that seen in association with arteriosclerosis or advanced cases of Raynaud's disease. It seems safe to conclude that, although some degree of conscious control over autonomic functions may be possible through biofeedback training, the control is partial and inconsistent. However, the therapeutic efficacy of biofeedback in treating migraine headaches is well established. It may be that short-lived changes in vascular tone, brought about by a combination of the relaxation component or skin temperature control through biofeedback, are sufficient to reverse the vasospasms and associated changes (in the absence of irreversible vascular pathology) that occur during a migraine episode.

Migraine is associated with intracranial vasoconstriction during the prodromal phase and with intra- and extracranial vasodilation during the headache phase [9–12]. Biofeedback-assisted hand-warming has been shown to be a phenomenon restricted to hands [13]; thus, it seems unlikely that vasodilation in the hands can reverse the migraine vasopathology of the cranial vessels directly. The relevance of hand-warming to migraine treatment is further questioned by the finding that about 70 to 80 percent of patients with migraine respond to biofeedback training in spite of the great intra- and interindividual variability in degrees of skin-temperature control obtained [14]. To date, no significant correlations have been demonstrated between degrees of skin-temperature change and migraine relief. The therapeutic efficacy of hand-warming, therefore, may involve another mechanism which in turn exerts some influence on intra- and extracranial blood flow. Sympathetic tone has been suggested, as it is closely related to both skin temperature and intra- and extracranial blood flow. Increases in sympathetic tone have been shown to decrease cutaneous blood flow and blood flow through the cranial vessels [15–20]. Relaxation procedures such as alpha enhancement, self-hypnosis, forehead electromyographic (EMG) feedback, autogenic relaxation training and transcendental meditation all possess antimigraine action [21–24]. The superiority of biofeedback-assisted hand-warming over the other relaxation techniques has not been demonstrated; in fact, EMG biofeedback training and Jacobson's relaxation technique were shown to be as effective as skin-temperature biofeedback in treating migraine headaches [25]. The available literature seems to suggest that the antimigraine element in biofeedback treatment is relaxation.

Increased activation of the sympathetic component of the autonomic nervous system frequently accompanies arousal, which forms the physiological basis for several emotions such as anxiety, anger, and excitement [26–28]. However, it has been pointed out that varying degrees of parasympathetic activation are also seen in association with arousal [29, 30]. Thus, since alterations in sympathetic activity are seldom seen in isolation, perhaps the term arousal should be used in place of sympathetic tone. Arousal is associated with a wide variety of physiological and biochemical changes in the body. Skin temperature alteration is only one of the peripheral physiological symptoms of arousal; changes in pulse rate, blood pressure, skin conductance, respiratory rate, etc., are also frequent accompaniments [31]. Mean amplitude and frequency of spontaneous fluctuation in skin conductance are considered by most experts as the most reliable index of arousal [31]. The logic, therefore, for choosing skin temperature instead of skin conductance for biofeedback training to reduce sympathetic tone or arousal is questionable.

Increases in epinephrine and norepinephrine are known to be related to stress. Earlier research suggested that a rise in epinephrine is characteristic of anxiety while an increase in norepinephrine is associated with anger, but subsequent studies failed to substantiate this. The current belief is that increases in plasma levels of both epinephrine and norepinephrine are characteristics of autonomic arousal, the physiological basis for a wide variety of mood changes [32–34]. Most epinephrine in peripheral blood is derived from the adrenal medulla; peripheral norepinephrine comes from postganglionic sympathetic nerve terminals [35].

Increased output of catecholamine metabolites has been reported during a migraine episode [36, 37]. Situations associated with arousal and increased catecholamine output, such as hypoglycemia, REM sleep, and premenstrual tension, have been linked to migraine headaches [38–40]. Similarly, tyramine, which releases norepinephrine from its binding sites, is well established as a migraine-evoking substance [40]. Some important biochemical changes that occur during the course of a migraine headache may be accounted for by increases in plasma catecholamines. Increase in free fatty acids accompanies arousal; these substances have been reported to cause platelet clumping with subsequent release of serotonin, which in turn leads to the prodromal phase of migraine headache characterized by vasoconstriction [38–44]. Presumably, a sudden drop in plasma serotonin triggers the headache phase of migraine [45, 46]. Since serotonin metabolism is carried out by monoamine oxidase (MAO), an increase in the activity of this enzyme seems to be required for the sudden fall in plasma serotonin accompanied by increased urinary excretion of its metabolite 5-HIAA [36, 47, 48]. Subcutaneous injections of epinephrine have been shown to elevate the activity of MAO in human beings some 15 to 20 minutes after the injection [49–51]. This delayed MAO response to catecholamines may be responsible for the drop in serotonin levels which is believed to underlie the headache phase of a migraine episode. The lowering of serotonin causes dilatation of extracranial blood vessels and a drop in central pain threshold [46].

We studied the effect of relaxation on catecholamine and monoamine oxidase levels, which seem relevant to migraine, in a group of patients with chronic anxiety.

METHOD

Twenty clinic patients, six men and 14 women (mean age 40.95 years; s.d. 11.53) diagnosed as having a generalized anxiety disorder (Research Diagnostic Criteria [52]) participated in the study. Twelve men and eight women (mean age 32.30; s.d. 6.91) were selected as a control group of physically and mentally healthy drug-free volunteers. A drug-free washout period of at least two weeks preceded the study. Physical examination of all subjects included T_3 and T_4 assays; special care was taken to rule out iron-deficiency anemia because this condition has been shown to influence platelet monoamine oxidase [53]. The subjects were instructed to avoid all forms of medication during the study period. Levels of anxiety were quantified by electromyograms (EMG) and with the State-Trait Anxiety Inventory [54] before biofeedback-assisted relaxation training began. Blood samples were drawn for biochemical assays before and after treatment, at the same time of day.

The State-Trait Anxiety Inventory consists of self-report scales that measure two distinct anxiety concepts, state anxiety and trait anxiety. State anxiety is seen as a transitory emotional condition of the human organism that is characterized by subjective, consciously perceived feelings of tension, apprehension, and heightened autonomic nervous system activity. Trait anxiety refers to differences in anxiety proneness, that is, variations between people in their tendency to respond to situations they perceive as threatening with intensified state anxiety [54].

For the next six weeks the subjects participated in 30- to 35-minute EMG biofeedback-assisted training sessions. Subjects were instructed to practice relaxation exercises at home for 20 minutes daily. After completing training, the subjects returned to the laboratory for final evaluation, according to the procedures outlined above.

Platelets were isolated from 12 ml of venous blood containing ACD solution and stored at $-80°$ C. Platelet counts were determined with a hemocytometer. Monoamine oxidase activity was assayed radiochemically using a modification of the procedure of Wurtman and Axelrod [55], with ^{14}C-tryptamine and ^{14}C-phenylethylamine as substrates. After the labeled products were extracted, aliquots were assayed for ^{14}C by liquid scintillation spectrometry and activity expressed as nmoles/product/4 $\times$ 10 platelets/hour.

For catecholamine assay blood samples were collected in vacutainer tubes containing EGTA and glutathione and immediately placed on ice. The sample was centrifuged at 1500 g for 10 minutes. Plasma was separated from the cells with a pipet, placed in a glass tube, and frozen immediaely at $-70°$ C. Catecholamine levels were estimated by a radioenzymatic thin-layer chromatographic technique based on the method of Peular and Johnson [56]. The assay used catecholamine-O-methyl transferase to convert the catecholamines to their O-methylated products. After separation by thin-layer chromatography, each labeled derivative was converted by peroxidase oxidation to the acid metabolite and extracted. Values were expressed as pg/ml. Biochemical assays of the pre- and post-treatment blood samples for both experimental and control groups were done at the same time after all samples were collected. Because of technical difficulties, catecholamines were assayed only for 15 subjects of the experimental group.

RESULTS

As catecholamine assays were available for 15 experimental subjects only, the first part of data analysis was done separately for monoamine

Table 1

Comparison of Pretreatment Psychological Measures and Enzyme Levels between Patients and Controls

Variable	Patients		Controls		t^*	p
	mean	s.d.	mean	s.d.		
State Anxiety ($n = 20$)	44.85	11.57	33.33	6.80	3.85	<.001
Trait Anxiety ($n = 20$)	51.70	8.58	31.55	7.20	8.04	<.001
Tryptamine ($n = 20$)	9.42	3.57	6.94	2.42	2.56	<.01
Phenylethylamine ($n = 20$)	37.26	14.33	29.29	10.79	1.99	<.05
Epinephrine ($n = 15$)	56.42	33.53	26.86	14.16	3.13	<.004
Norepinephrine ($n = 15$)	514.50	299.45	232.26	81.53	3.52	<.002

* two-tail t-test
MAO (PEA and trypt) expressed as nmoles/4 × 10^8/hr.
Epinephrine and norepinephrine expressed as pg/ml.

oxidase activity and catecholamines. Subjects were six men and nine women with a mean age of 38.26, s.d. 12.03. Controls were seven men and eight women with a mean age of 32.82, s.d. 7.92. Index and control groups were compared via t-test based on pretreatment data (Table 1).

Table 2 presents changes in anxiety scores and biochemical values following relaxation training. Pearson product-moment correlations were calculated between monoamine oxidase and catecholamine levels before and after treatment (Tables 3 and 4).

DISCUSSION

The results indicated reduced epinephrine, norepinephrine, and monoamine oxidase levels after biofeedback-assisted relaxation training. Significant correlations were found between plasma catecholamine and monoamine oxidase levels, before and after relaxation training. There is some uncertainty whether these biochemical changes are specifically related to anxiety or are mainly due to nonspecific factors. Venipuncture, for example, has been shown to elevate plasma levels of catecholamines; it may be argued, then, that the biochemical changes represent the patients' response to venipuncture and not resting anxiety levels [57, 58]. Similarly, the decrease in catecholamine values after treatment may be the result of patients' habituation to the venipuncture procedure rather than a decrease in anxiety. Blood samples were drawn after 35 minutes

Table 2

Pre- and Post-treatment Changes of Psychological Measures and Enzyme Levels in Patients and Controls

	mean	s.d.	mean	s.d.	t*	p	mean	s.d.	mean	s.d.	t*	p
State Anxiety ($n = 20$)	44.85	11.57	32.20	6.68	5.21	<.001	33.30	6.80	34.50	12.29	0.55	NS
Trait Anxiety ($n = 20$)	51.70	8.58	40.60	10.31	5.50	<.001	31.55	7.20	33.35	10.88	1.18	NS
Tryptamine ($n = 20$)	9.42	3.57	7.66	2.25	3.34	<.003	6.94	2.42	7.05	2.77	0.48	NS
Phenylethylamine ($n = 20$)	37.26	14.33	32.10	10.42	2.42	<.03	29.29	10.79	29.36	11.80	0.08	NS
Epinephrine ($n = 20$)	56.42	33.53	39.00	20.27	2.49	<.03	26.86	14.16	32.06	24.80	1.13	NS
Norepinephrine ($n = 15$)	514.50	299.45	402.71	210.51	2.18	<.05	232.26	81.53	223.93	50.92	0.48	NS
EMG ($n = 15$)	3.20	2.02	1.21	0.60	4.28	<.001						

* paired t-test

Table 3

Correlation between Pre Scores on Psychological and Biochemical Data (Patients $n = 15$)

	State Anxiety	Trait Anxiety	EMG	Tryptamine	Phenylethylamine	Epinephrine	Norepinephrine
State Anxiety	—	.71***	.32	.39	.48	.20	.23
Trait Anxiety	—	—	.38	.09	.18	.04	.18
EMG	—	—	—	.11	.17	.06	.01
Tryptamine	—	—	—	—	.98***	.46**	.50**
Phenylethylamine	—	—	—	—	—	.46**	.49**
Epinephrine	—	—	—	—	—	—	.24

*** $p < .001$
** $p < .05$

of relaxation in a semidark room, and the procedure was discussed with the patients in advance; none of the subjects exhibited an excessive fear of the procedure. Participants' electromyographic and skin conductance responses were monitored during this period, and no increase in anxiety level during venipuncture was noted. In spite of all the precautions, the effect of trauma associated with venipuncture cannot be ruled out.

The observed biochemical changes cannot be attributed to circadian alterations in plasma catecholamines and monoamine oxidase as blood samples were drawn at the same time of the day for both index and control groups [59, 60]. Spontaneous fluctuations may account for changes

Table 4

Correlation between Post Scores on Psychological and Biochemical Data (Patients $n = 15$)

	State Anxiety	Trait Anxiety	EMG	Tryptamine	Phenylethylamine	Epinephrine	Norepinephrine
State Anxiety	—	.82**	.01	.07	.09	.09	.09
Trait Anxiety	—	—	.03	.04	.01	.14	.01
EMG	—	—	—	.00	.00	.18	.02
Tryptamine	—	—	—	—	.97***	.54**	.31
Phenylethylamine	—	—	—	—	—	.51**	.30
Epinephrine	—	—	—	—	—	—	.26

*** $p < .001$
** $p < .05$

in catecholamines, but in normal subjects monoamine oxidase activity is known to remain stable over long periods [61]. Dietary factors and physical exertion have been shown to influence plasma catecholamine levels [32]. Since the blood samples were drawn after 35 minutes of relaxation, however, the effect of exercise is unlikely. Dietary factors were not controlled. Although the index and control groups were not age-matched, no significant differences were present between the two. Menstruation is another possible explanation for the alterations in biochemical values [32, 61].

An important finding of the study is the significant decrease in platelet monoamine oxidase following relaxation and the correlation between plasma catecholamines and platelet monoamine oxidase. Our results substantiate a previous report on the effect of relaxation on monoamine oxidase [62]. Evidence from other sources also supports a relationship between anxiety and monoamine oxidase activity. Stress has been shown to increase the activity of this enzyme in animals [63]. Similarly, an association between stress-related hormones, such as ACTH and adrenalin, and MAO has been demonstrated [49, 50, 51, 64]. Although our findings indicate a significant correlation between plasma catecholamines and monoamine oxidase activity, the precise nature of the relationship is uncertain. Epinephrine may directly affect monoamine oxidase, or the relationship may involve the intervention of a third stress-related hormone such as ACTH or thyroxine.

The present findings suggest that biofeedback-assisted relaxation may reduce plasma levels of catecholamines and platelet monoamine oxidase activity. Reduction in catecholamines during the prodrome of migraine may prevent the release of free fatty acids, platelet clumping, release of serotonin from platelets, release of prostaglandins and other vasoactive substances. Increase in plasma serotonin levels is prevented by decrease in monoamine oxidase activity with stabilization of plasma serotonin levels.

The hypothesis has some weaknesses. The biochemical explanation for the antimigraine effect of biofeedback presented here is based on the serotonin theory of migraine, which is not universally accepted. Increase in monoamine oxidase activity in migraine has not been demonstrated; in fact decreases have been reported [65]. The present findings were found on Type B platelet monoamine oxidase which has no action on serotonin substrate. To what extent these findings can be generalized to Type A enzyme which has a more specific action on serotonin [66], is uncertain. Finally, it is questionable whether these results, based on anxious subjects, can be applied to patients suffering from migraine.

REFERENCES

1. Board of Directors, American Association for the Study of Headache: Biofeedback therapy. *Headache* 18:107, 1978.
2. Sargent JD, Green EE, Walters ED: The use of autogenic feedback training in a pilot study of migraine and tension headaches. *Headache* 12:120–125, 1972.
3. Wickramasekera IE: Temperature feedback for the control of migraine. *Journal of Behavior Therapy and Experimental Psychiatry* 4:343–345, 1973.
4. Fahrion SL: Autogenic biofeedback treatment for migraine. *Mayo Clin Proc* 52: 776–784, 1977.
5. Benson H: *The Relaxation Response*. New York, Avon Books, 1975.
6. Wallace RK: Physiological effects of transcendental meditation. *Science* 167:1751–1754, 1970.
7. Wallace RK, Benson H: Physiology of meditation, in *Altered States of Awareness—Readings from Scientific American*. San Francisco, WH Freedman & Company, 1972.
8. Dicara LV: Learning in the autonomic nervous system, in *Altered States of Awareness—Readings from Scientific American*. San Francisco, WH Freedman & Company, 1972.
9. Norris JW, Hachinski VC, Cooper PW: Changes in cerebral blood flow during a migraine attack. *Br Med J* 3:676–684, 1975.
10. Mathew NT, Hrastnik F, Meyer JS: Regional cerebral blood flow in the diagnosis of vascular headache. *Headache* 15:252–260, 1976.
11. Edmeads J: Cerebral blood flow in migraine. *Headache* 17:148–152, 1977.
12. Sakai F, Meyer JS: Regional cerebral hemodynamics during migraine and cluster headaches measured by the ^{133}Xe inhalation method. *Headache* 18:122–132, 1978.
13. Taub E: Self-regulation of human tissue temperature, in Schwartz GE, Beatty J (eds): *Biofeedback Theory and Research*. New York, Academic Press, 1977.
14. Diamond S, Medina JL: The treatment of headache with different modalities of biofeedback therapy (abstract). *Headache* 16:80–81, 1976.
15. Brod J: Circulation in muscle during acute pressor responses to emotional stress and during chronic sustained elevation of blood pressure. *Am Heart J* 68:424–426, 1974.
16. Sokolov YN: *Percentage and Conditioned Reflex*. New York, Macmillan, 1963.
17. Nagai H, Mahe H, Furuse M, Takagai T: The role of sympathetic nerve and vasoactive amines in cerebral vasospasm, in Ingvar DH, Lassen NA (eds): *Cerebral Function Metabolism and Circulation*. *Acta Neurol Scand* 56 (Suppl 64), 1977.
18. Kawamura Y, Meyer JS, Hiromoto H, Aoyagi M, Hashi K: Neurogenic control of cerebral blood flow in the baboon. *J Neurosurg* 43:676–688, 1975.
19. Kobayashi S, Wallz AG, Rhoton AL: Effects of stimulation of cervical sympathetic nerves on cortical blood flow and vascular reactivity. *Neurology* 21:297–302, 1971.

20. Harper AM, Deshmukh VD, Rowan JO, Jennett WB: The influence of sympathetic nervous activity on cerebral blood flow. *Arch Neurol* 27:1-6, 1972.
21. Andreychuk T, Skriver C: Hypnosis and biofeedback in the treatment of migraine headache. *Int J Clin Exp Hypn* 23:172-183, 1975.
22. Bakal DA, Kaganov JA: Muscle contraction and migraine headache: Psychophysiological comparison. *Headache* 17:208-215, 1977.
23. Luthe W: Autogenic training: Method, research and application in medicine. *Am J Psychiatry* 17:174-195, 1963.
24. Benson H, Maluea BP, Graham JR: Physiologic correlates of meditation and their clinical effects in headache: An ongoing investigation. *Headache* 13:23-24, 1973.
25. Blanchard EB, Theobald DE, Williamson DA, Silver BV, Brown DA: Temperature biofeedback in the treatment of migraine headaches. *Arch Gen Psychiatry* 35:581-588, 1978.
26. Duffy E: Activation, in Greenfield NS and Sternbach RA (eds): *Handbook of Psychophysiology*. New York, Holt, Rinehart and Winston, 1972.
27. Martin B: The assessment of anxiety by physiological behavioral measures. *Psychol Bull* 58:234-255, 1961.
28. Schacter S, Singer JE: Cognitive, social and physiological determinants of emotional state. *Psychol Rev* 69:379-399, 1962.
29. Gellhorn E, Kiely WF: Autonomic nervous system in psychiatric disorder, in Mendels J (ed): *Biological Psychiatry*. New York, Wiley-Interscience, 1973.
30. Kiely WF: From the symbolic stimulus to the pathophysiological response: Neurophysiological mechanisms, in Lipowski ZT, Lipsitt DR, Whybrow PC (eds): *Psychosomatic Medicine*. New York, Oxford University Press, 1977.
31. Lader MH: Psychophysiology of anxiety, in Lader MH (ed): *Studies of Anxiety*. Ashford, Kent, Headley Brothers, 1969.
32. Levi L: Stress and distress in response to psychosocial stimuli. *Acta Med Scand* 191, Suppl 528, 1968.
33. Mason JW: A review of psychoendocrine research in the sympathetic adrenal medullary system. *Psychosom Med* 30:631-653, 1968.
34. Frankenheuser M: Experimental approaches to the study of catecholamines and emotions, in Levi L (ed): *Emotions: Their Parameters and Measurements*. New York, Raven Press, 1975.
35. Carrier O Jr.: *Pharmacology of the Peripheral Autonomic Nervous System*. Chicago, Yearbook Medical Publishers, 1972.
36. Curran DA, Hinterberger H, Lance JW: Total plasma serotonin, 5-hydroxy indole acetic acid, and 4-hydroxy-3-methoxy mandelic acid excretion in normal migraine subjects. *Brain* 88:997-1010, 1965.
37. Lance JW, Anthony M, Hinterberger H: The control of cranial arteries by hormonal mechanisms and its relation to migraine syndrome. *Headache* 7:93-102, 1967.
38. Hockaday JM, Williamson DH, Whitty CWM: Blood glucose levels and fatty acid metabolism in migraine related to fasting. *Lancet* 1:1153-1156, 1971.
39. Rees L: Stress, distress and disease. *Br J Psychiatry* 128:3-19, 1976.

40. Lance JW: *Mechanism and Management of Headache.* London, Butterworths, 1978.
41. Levi L: Neuroendocrinology of anxiety, in Lader MH (ed): *Studies of Anxiety.* Ashford, Kent, Headley Brothers, 1969.
42. Anthony M: The role of free fatty acids in migraine. Presented to First International Migraine Symposium, London, England, 1977.
43. Silver MH, Smith JB, Ingerman C: Arachidonic acid induced human platelet aggregation and prostaglandin formation. *Prostaglandins* 4:863–875, 1973.
44. Deshmukh SV, Meyer JS: Cyclic changes in platelet dynamics and the pathogenesis and prophylaxis of migraine. *Headache* 17:101–108, 1977.
45. Franchamps A: The role of humoral mediators in migraine headache. *Can J Neurol Sci* 1:189–195, 1979.
46. Anthony M, Lance JW: The role of serotonin in migraine, in Pearce J (ed): *Modern Topics in Migraine.* London, Heinemann, 1975.
47. Cooper JR, Bloom FE, Roth RH: *The Biochemical Basis of Neuropharmacology.* New York, Oxford University Press, 1978.
48. Sicuteri F, Testi A, Anselmi B: Biochemical investigations in headache: Increases in hydroxy indole acetic acid excretion during attacks. *Int Arch Allergy Appl Immunol* 19:55–58, 1961.
49. Gentil V, Greenwood MH, Lader MH: The effect of adrenalin on human platelet MAO activity. *Psychopharmacologia (Berlin)* 44:187–190, 1975.
50. Gentil V, McCurdy RL, Alevizos A, Laden MH: The effect of adrenalin injections on human platelet monoamine oxidase and releated measures. *Psychopharmacology* 50:187–192, 1976.
51. Owen F, Acker W, Bourne RC, Frith CD, and Riley GJ: The effect on human monoamine oxidase activity of subcutaneous injections of adrenalin. *Biochem Pharmacol* 26:2065–2067, 1977.
52. Spitzer R, Endicott J, Robins E: *Research Diagnostic Criteria for a Selected Group of Functional Disorders.* New York, New York Psychiatric Institute Biometric Research Division, 1975.
53. Callender S, Graham-Smith DG, Woods HF: Reduction of platelet monoamine oxidase activity in iron deficiency anaemea. *Br J Pharmacol* 52:447–448, 1974.
54. Spielberger CD, Gorsuch RL, Lushene RD: *STAI Manual.* Palo Alto, Consulting Psychologists Press, 1970.
55. Wurtman RT, Axelrod J: A sensitive and specific assay for the estimation of monoamine oxidase. *Biochem Pharmacol* 12:1439–1440, 1963.
56. Peular JD, Johnson GA: A sensitive radioimmunoassay of plasma catecholamines: Initial studies in supine normotensive subjects. *Clin Res* 23:474, 1975.
57. Lake CR, Ziegler MG, Kopin IJ: Use of plasma norepinephrine for evaluation of sympathetic neuronal function in man. *Life Sci* 18:1315–1326, 1976.
58. Carruthers M, Conway N, Taggart P, Convay N, Bates D: Validity of plasma catecholamine estimations. *Lancet* 1:62–67, 1970.
59. Aronow WS, Harding PR, DeQuattro V, Isbell M: Diurnal variation of plasma catecholamines and systolic time intervals. *Chest* 63:722–726, 1973.

60. Akerstedt T: Altered sleep/wake patterns and circadian rhythms. *Acta Physiol Scand* (Suppl 469), 1979.
61. Murphy DL, Wright C, Buchsbaum M, Nichols A, Costa JL, Wyatt RJ: Platelet and plasma amine oxidase activity in 680 normals: Sex and age differences over time. *Biochem Med* 16:254–265, 1976.
62. Mathew RJ, Ho BT, Kralik P, Claghorn JL: Biochemical basis for biofeedback treatment of migraine: A hypothesis. *Headache*: 19:290–293, 1979.
63. Maura G, Versace P, Paudice P: Chronic environmental stress on the development of MAO and COMT in discrete brain regions. *Pharmacol Res Commun* 10: 235–241, 1978.
64. Bhagat B, Bryan RJ, Lee YC: Increase in adrenal monoamine oxidase activity in hypophysectomized rats after ACTH. *Neuropharmacology* 12:1199–1202, 1973.
65. Sandler M: Monoamines and migraine: A path through the woods, in Diamond S, Dalessio DJ, Graham JR (eds): *Vasoactive Substances Relevant to Migraine*. Springfield, Ill, Charles C Thomas, 1975.
66. Donnelly C, Murphy DL: Substrate and inhibitor related characteristics of human platelet monoamine oxidase. *Biochem Pharmacol* 26:853–858, 1977.

Chapter 9

Evaluation of Relaxation Training as Treatment for Migraine Headaches

EDWARD B. BLANCHARD, Ph.D.
TIM A. AHLES

Sparked by the work of Sargent, Green, and their colleagues on the use of "autogenic feedback training" [1, 2], scientists of the 1970s have witnessed a tremendous outpouring of research on the various psychological treatments for migraine headaches. These treatments included several varieties of relaxation training.

Although the rationale for using relaxation training with migraine headaches has rarely been made explicit, the implicit rationale seems to be tied to the ideas that a migraine headache is mediated to some extent by sympathetic nervous system arousal and that relaxation training can reduce the level of sympathetic arousal. Hence, the hope that regular practice of some form of relaxation may be prophylactic for migraine.

In this paper we will do two things: First, we will summarize and evaluate the research on treatment of migraine headache solely with relaxation training. Second, we will compare the results from studies in which relaxation training alone has been used with results from two other popular psychological treatments, temperature biofeedback training alone, and the combination of temperature biofeedback training and autogenic training, using a new analytic procedure called meta-analysis.

RELAXATION TRAINING AND MIGRAINE

Bases for Evaluation

Relaxation techniques

We have chosen to define relaxation training broadly and thus have included studies in which the relaxation training was an abbreviated form of Jacobson's progressive relaxation training [3], made popular by Wolpe [4] and Paul [5], in which the major muscle groups of the body are alternately tensed and relaxed; a passive, meditative form of relaxation, epitomized by Benson's regular elicitation of the "relaxation response" [6]; the use of frontal electromyographic (EMG) biofeedback training as a general relaxation technique [7]; and hypnosis, which uses a relaxation induction technique. Reports which have used any of these forms of relaxation training will be included in this analysis.

Experimental design

The first consideration in evaluating a treatment procedure, in our opinion, must be efficacy. Does the treatment work? The strength of these conclusions is determined by both the results obtained and the design of the experiment. In previous reports [8, 9] we have described a hierarchy of experimental designs; the higher the hierarchy, the more confidence one could have in the results. These designs, in ascending order, are anecdotal case report, systematic case study, single group (uncontrolled) outcome study, single subject experiment, and controlled group outcome study. We shall use this same system.

In considering the treatment of headache, there is a second aspect of efficacy which should be considered, efficacy along the dimension of headache complaints. Thus one needs to consider, at a minimum, frequency, duration, intensity of the pain, and probably medication consumption.

Other evaluation bases

As one of us (Blanchard) has pointed out elsewhere [9], there are aspects of evaluation other than efficacy. These include efficiency, or how rapidly the treatment works; generality, or for what percentage of an unselected patient population the treatment is effective; and durability, or how well the treatment effects hold up over time—or, put another way, follow-up.

Finally, given some of the ambiguity present in the diagnosis or classification of headache [10], one needs to consider whether the patient sample was appropriate for a study of migraine headache. The best way to determine this is if the study gives explicit inclusion and exclusion criteria so that one can be certain that the patients were suffering from migraine headaches.

Summary of Previous Research

Tables 1 and 2 list the studies we could identify which used some form of relaxation training as the only specified treatment for a group of migraine patients. We have adopted the convention of calculating a percentage of improvement for each of the potential dimensions of efficacy, using the following formula:

$$\frac{\text{baseline value} - \text{end of treatment value}}{\text{baseline value}} \times 100 = \text{percentage improvement}$$

Only those studies published in archival sources by September 1979 were included.

Several observations are readily apparent from examining the tables. First, there are several conspicuous gaps in the tables, indicating missing data. This is especially the case in terms of follow-up information: although five of seven studies provide some kind of follow-up information at either three or six months, in only one case [16] is one-year follow-up available. The topic of selection criteria is also somewhat wanting as only two studies give specific criteria. Finally, there are no data on treatment efficiency.

The results on treatment efficacy range from virtually no improvement, at least at the end of treatment [14], to as high as 100 percent [17]. (This last value seems inflated in that only a 33-percent reduction in symptoms was required for a patient to be rated as improved by Lake and his colleagues [17].) In six of the seven studies, some degree of improvement was found as a result of relaxation training alone. (This high percentage of positive results could be a function of journal editorial policy of only publishing positive findings, however.)

One question we have sought to answer is: What is the best estimate of the degree of improvement one can expect from the treatment of migraine headache by relaxation training alone? Unfortunately, results for no single dependent variable appear in all reports. Therefore, we have taken the somewhat unorthodox step of averaging two different variables: the headache index when it was available and the percentage of the sam-

Table 1
Summary of Studies Using Relaxation Training to Treat Migraine Headache

Author(s)	No. of Pts. in Relax. Condition	Selection Criteria	Type of Relaxation Training	Duration of Baseline	Duration of Training	Experiment Design	Other Conditions
Hay, Madders (1971) [11]	98	Dx. by neurologist	Abbrev. progressive relaxation (Group)	None	6 wks (1/wk)	Single group outcome	
Warner, Lance (1975) [12]	14	Referred by neurologist	Abbrev. progressive relaxation (indiv.)	None	4 wks (1/wk)	Single group outcome	
Benson, Klemchuk, Graham (1974) [13]	17	N/A	TM	1–3 months	4 days	Single group outcome	
Mitchell, Mitchell (1971) [14]	7	Dx. migraine	Abbrev. progressive relaxation (indiv.)	8 wks	8 wks (2/wk)	Controlled group outcome	1. No trt. 2. Comb. desens. (C.D.)
Andreychuk, Skriver (1975) [15]	10	N/A	Hypnosis & relaxation	6 wks	10 wks (1/wk)	Controlled group outcome	1. Alpha biofeedback 2. Temp. biofeedback + autogenic trng.
Blanchard et al. (1978) [16]	13	Specific inclusion & exclusion	Abbrev. progressive relaxation (indiv.)	1 month	6 wks (2/wk)	Controlled group outcome	1. No trt. 2. Temp. biofeedback + autogenic trng.
Lake, Rainey, Papsdorf (1979) [17]	6	Specific inclusion criteria	Frontal EMG biofeedback	4 wks	4 wks (2/wk)	Controlled group outcome	1. No trt. 2. Temp. biofeedback

Notes: N/A, information not available in article; R, relaxation condition; TM, Transcendental Meditation.

Table 2

Summary of Results of Studies Using Relaxation Training to Treat Migraine

Author(s)	Results—End of Treatment			Follow-up Results Percentage Improvement		
	Efficacy		Generality (% sample improved)	3 mo.	6 mo.	1 yr.
	Percentage Improvement	Relative Efficacy				
Hay, Madders (1971) [11]	—	—	70%	None	—	—
Warner, Lance (1975) [12]	—	—	—	—	83% of Ss were improved by at least 50% in frequency	—
Benson, Klemchuk, Graham (1974) [13]	HA Index—16%	—	18%	35% of Ss were rated improved	—	—
Mitchell, Mitchell (1970) [14]	HA Index—N/A F—0% I—N/A D—0% Meds—N/A	R = No Trt. CD > R	N/A	—	(8 mo) HA Index—N/A F—24% I—N/A D—0 Meds—N/A % Ss improved 43%	—

Table 2 (continued)
Summary of Results of Studies Using Relaxation Training to Treat Migraine

Author(s)	Results—End of Treatment			Follow-up Results Percentage Improvement		
	Efficacy		Generality (% sample improved)	3 mo.	6 mo.	1 yr.
	Percentage Improvement	Relative Efficacy				
Andreychuk, Skriver (1975) [15]	HA Index—37%*	R = Temp. BFD R = Alpha BFD	N/A	None	—	—
Blanchard et al. [16]	HA Index—81%* F—68%* I—56%* D—67%* Meds—54%*	R > No Trt. R > Temp. BFD	85%	HA Index—45%* F—68%* I—41%* D—88%* Meds—29% 56% of sample still markedly improved R = Temp. BFD	—	HA Index—83%* F—50%* I—51%* D—87%* Meds—88%* R = Temp. BFD
Lake, Rainey, Papsdorf (1979) [17]	HA Index—26%* F—N/A I—N/A D—N/A Meds—N/A	R = Temp. BFD R > No Trt.	100% (at 33% improved)	HA Index—52%* F—* I—* D—* Meds—N/A	—	—

Notes: * Indicates significant within-group improvement; HA Index, composite headache index; F, frequency; I, intensity; D, duration; Meds, medication consumption.

ple judged to be improved in the absence of a value for headache index. This yields an estimate of 38.3-percent improvement at the end of treatment ($n = 6$), and 51.6-percent improvement at follow-ups of three to six months ($n = 5$).

As to relative efficacy, in two of three cases treatment by relaxation was significantly better than no treatment. In only one instance, however, was relaxation training better than any other form of psychological treatment: Blanchard et al. [16] found treatment by abbreviated, progressive relaxation superior to temperature biofeedback combined with autogenic training at the end of the six-week training period. This difference was no longer statistically significant at follow-ups of one, three, or 12 months. Thus, there is no basis in terms of efficacy for choosing relaxation training over any other form of psychological treatment.

Looking at the percentage of patients in the sample who were improved, either at the end of treatment or during follow-up, we find values ranging from 35 percent to 100 percent, with a mean value ($n = 6$) of 64.5 percent. It would appear that two of every three migraine patients treated by relaxation training improve to some extent.

Since relaxation training can easily be administered to groups by a paraprofessional staff member, and even by self-instructional tapes, it may prove to be a very cost-effective treatment for migraine headaches.

COMPARISON OF RELAXATION TRAINING AND THERMAL BIOFEEDBACK IN THE TREATMENT OF MIGRAINE

As was mentioned earlier, one of the principal factors of the increased interest in treatment of migraine headache by psychological means was the work of the Menninger group on the use of combined thermal biofeedback training and autogenic training. We shall compare the results obtained in treating migraine headache with relaxation training to those obtained with thermal biofeedback alone and thermal biofeedback combined with autogenic training.

Stroebel and Glueck [18] have suggested that biofeedback may be the "ultimate placebo." In an effort to determine if the treatment effects obtained with the various psychological techniques can be dismissed solely as placebo effects, the results from the three previously mentioned psychological treatments will be compared with results obtained with a standard pharmacological placebo. We have omitted the work on cephalic vasomotor biofeedback [19, 20] because of a lack of data, except from Friar and Beatty [19] on groups of patients treated with this technique.

Bases for Comparison

In this type of comparison, known as a meta-analysis [21, 22], the results for a whole group of subjects given a particular treatment become the units of analysis. The data we have used in this study for the thermal biofeedback studies are summarized in Table 3.

In conducting this type of analysis, certain *a priori* conditions must be set. Thus we included studies which were either single group outcome

Table 3

Summary of Results of Treatment by Thermal Biofeedback Alone or with Autogenic Training

Authors	Conditions	# Pts.	End of Treatment		3–6 Mo. Follow-Up	
			% Improv. in HA Index	% Sample Improved	% Improv. in HA Index	% Sample Improved
Sargent et al. (1972) [1]	TBFD + AT	62	—	74	—	—
Sargent et al. (1973) [2]	TBFD + AT	19	—	63	—	—
Reading, Mohr (1976) [23]	TBFD + AT	6	40	—	66	—
Fried et al. (1977) [24]	TBFD + AT	5	—	60	—	—
Fahrion (1977) [25]	TBFD + AT	21	—	—	—	71
Blanchard et al. (1978) [16]	TBFD + AT	13	73	54	63	40
	No Trt.	10	23	10	—	—
Turin, Johnson (1976) [26]	TBFD	7	41	57	—	—
Mullinix et al. (1978) [27]	TBFD	6	21	63	—	—
	Control	5	8	—	—	—
Andreychuk, Skriver (1975) [15]	TBFD	9	82	—	—	—
Mitch et al. (1976) [28]	TBFD	20	—	75	—	80
Largen et al. (1979) [29]	TBFD	13		83		
Lake et al. (1979) [17]	TBFD	6	32	—	32	—
	No Trt.	6	17	—	−4	—

Notes: TBFD, thermal biofeedback
AT, autogenic training

or controlled group outcome and had a minimum of five subjects in a treatment condition of interest. To arrive at a value for the degree of improvement, we followed the same convention we used in the earlier part of this article: when the data were provided, we calculated a percentage improvement score for a global headache index. When this value could not be obtained, we used a value for the percentage of the sample judged to be clinically improved. Finally, we used the results from the end of treatment when these were available; however, in the absence of these data (see Table 3), we used a value from a follow-up of three or six months. All these steps were taken, of course, to increase the sample size for analysis.

To determine a value for the placebo response of migraine headache, we took comparable improvement scores from studies in which an active drug was compared to a placebo in a double-blind controlled trial. Only those studies in which an estimate of treatment response to placebo could be obtained (hence these were available either as pretreatment headache activity data or as a score on degree of improvement from pretreatment state) were included in the analysis. The values for placebo response are summarized in Table 4.

Interestingly, the average value for the three groups of subjects who received no treatment [14, 16, 17] was 13.4 percent, very close to the mean value for placebo shown in Table 4.

Results of Meta-Analysis

The values from Tables 1–4 were subjected to a one-way analysis of variance. This yielded mean improvement scores of: relaxation alone—50.9, temperature biofeedback alone—55.7, temperature biofeedback combined with autogenic training—63.5, and placebo—16.5. The initial anal-

Table 4

Effects of Placebo on Migraine Headache

Authors	Sample Size	Percentage Improvement from Placebo
Lance et al. (1970) [30]	50	32
Waters (1970) [10]	79	18
Weber, Reinmuth (1972) [31]	19	11
Ludvigsson (1974) [32]	32	25
Vardi et al. (1976) [33]	26	0
Kallanranta et al. (1977) [34]	20	13

$x = 16.5\%$

ysis yielded a significant overall between-groups effect ($F = 5.64$, $df = 3,21$, $p = 0.0054$). Further individual comparisons showed that each of the treatment conditions yielded significantly more improvement than placebo ($p = 0.005$ or less). However, the t values for pairwise comparisons among the three treatment conditions were all less than 1.0, indicating no significant difference between any pair of conditions.

Power analysis

Because of the way the hypotheses are stated in analysis of variance, we may either reject the null hypothesis of "no difference among the conditions" or not be able to reject it. Not being able to reject the null hypothesis, however, is not equivalent to accepting it. To determine if our calculated lack of difference truly reflects no difference, we must perform a power analysis.

Following the procedures described by Keppel [35], we calculated the power of the comparison of relaxation alone, temperature biofeedback alone, and temperature biofeedback combined with autogenic training. Setting the α (alpha) level at 0.05, the observed power $(1 - \beta)$ (beta) is 0.81. This means β is equal to 0.19, or that there is only about one chance in five that, if differences existed among the treatments, their detection would not have occurred in this analysis.

DISCUSSION

This paper has summarized the results obtained from several studies of the treatment of migraine headache with various forms of relaxation. The average response of several groups of patients treated with relaxation was compared to the average response to a placebo medication and found to be significantly better; it was also compared to the average response to treatment by temperature biofeedback and found to be equivalent. The three direct experimental comparisons [15, 16, 17] yield similar results. This latter finding implies that, on the basis of cost, one might choose relaxation over biofeedback.

There is further temptation to speculate that temperature biofeedback training may operate by the same mechanism as relaxation, since they have equivalent results. It could be that both operate through some final common pathway. The studies and analyses presented in this paper, however, neither support nor deny such a speculation. Further research is required.

ACKNOWLEDGMENT

Preparation of this manuscript was supported in part by a grant from the National Institute of Neurological and Communicative Disorders and Stroke, NS-15235-01. The authors thank Drs. Frank Andrasik and Dennis O'Keefe for their assistance on parts of this paper.

REFERENCES

1. Sargent JD, Green EE, Walters ED: The use of autogenic feedback training in a pilot study of migraine and tension headaches. *Headache* 12:120–125, 1972.
2. Sargent JD, Green EE, Walters ED: Preliminary report on the use of autogenic feedback training in the treatment of migraine and tension headaches. *Psychosom Med* 35:129–135, 1973.
3. Jacobson E: The technique of progressive relaxation. *J Nerv Ment Dis* 60:568–578, 1924.
4. Wolpe J: *Psychotherapy by Reciprocal Inhibition*. Stanford, Cal., Stanford University Press, 1958.
5. Paul GL: *Insight vs. Desensitization in Psychotherapy: An Experiment in Anxiety Reduction*. Stanford, Cal., Stanford University Press, 1966.
6. Benson H: *The Relaxation Response*. New York, Morrow, 1975.
7. Stoyva J, Budzynski T: Cultivated low arousal—an antistress response?, in Dicara LV (ed): *Limbic and Autonomic Nervous Systems Research*. New York, Plenum, 1974.
8. Blanchard EB, Young LD: Clinical applications of biofeedback training: A review of evidence. *Arch Gen Psychiatry* 30:573–589, 1974.
9. Blanchard EB: Biofeedback and the modification of cardiovascular dysfunctions, in Gatchel RJ, Price KP (eds): *Clinical Applications of Biofeedback: Appraisal and Status*. New York, Pergamon, 1979.
10. Waters WE: Controlled clinical trial of ergotamine tartrate. *Br Med J* 2:325–327, 1970.
11. Hay KM, Madders J: Migraine treated by relaxation therapy. *J R Coll Gen Pract* 21:664–749, 1971.
12. Warner G, Lance JW: Relaxation therapy in migraine and chronic tension headache. *Med J Aust* 1:298–301, 1975.
13. Benson H, Klemchuk, HP, Graham, JR: The usefulness of the relaxation response in the therapy of headache. *Headache* 14:49–52, 1974.
14. Mitchell KR, Mitchell DM: Migraine: An exploratory treatment application of programmed behavior therapy technique. *J Psychsom Res* 15:137–157, 1971.
15. Andreychuk T, Skriver C: Hypnosis and biofeedback in the treatment of migraine headache. *Int J Clin Exp Hypn* 23:172–183, 1975.
16. Blanchard EB, Theobald DE, Williamson DA, Silver BV, Brown DA: Temperature biofeedback in the treatment of migraine headaches. *Arch Gen Psychiatry* 35:581–588, 1978.

17. Lake A, Raney J, Papsdorf JD: Biofeedback and rational-emotive therapy in the management of migraine headache. *J Appl Behav Anal* 12:127–140, 1979.
18. Stroebel CF, Glueck BC: Biofeedback treatment in medicine and psychiatry: An ultimate placebo? in Birk L (ed): *Biofeedback: Behavioral Medicine*. New York, Grune & Stratton, 1973.
19. Friar LR, Beatty J: Migraine: Management by trained control of vasoconstriction. *J Consult Clin Psychol* 44:46–53, 1976.
20. Feuerstein M, Adams HE: Cephalic vasomotor feedback in the modification of migraine headache. *Biofeedback Self Regul* 2:241–254, 1977.
21. Glass GV: Primary, secondary, and meta-analysis of research. *Educational Researcher* 10:3–8, 1976.
22. Smith ML, Glass GV: Meta-analysis of psychotherapy outcome studies. *Am Psychol* 32:752–760, 1977.
23. Reading C, Mohr PD: Biofeedback control of migraine: A pilot study. *Br J Soc Clin Psychol* 15:429–433, 1976.
24. Fried FE, Lambert J, Sneed P: Treatment of tension and migraine headaches with biofeedback techniques. *Mo Med* 74:253–255, 1977.
25. Fahrion SL: Autogenic biofeedback treatment for migraine. *Mayo Clin Proc* 52:776–784, 1977.
26. Turin A, Johnson WG: Biofeedback therapy for migraine headaches. *Arch Gen Psychiatry* 33:517–519, 1976.
27. Mullinix J, Norton B, Hack S, Fishman M: Skin temperature biofeedback and migraine. *Headache* 17:242–244, 1978.
28. Mitch PS, McGrady A, Iannone A: Autogenic feedback training in migraine: A treatment report. *Headache* 15:267–270, 1976.
29. Largen JW, Mathew RJ, Dobbins K, Meyer JS, Sakai F, Claghorn JL: The effect of direction of skin temperature self-regulation on migraine activity and regional cerebral blood flow, in *Proceedings of the Biofeedback Society of America 10th Annual Meeting*. Denver, Biofeedback Society of America, 1979. pp 76–78.
30. Lance JW, Anthony M, Somerville B: Comparative trial of serotonin antagonists in the management of migraine. *Br Med J* 2:327–330, 1970.
31. Weber RB, Reinmuth O: The treatment of migraine with propranolol. *Neurology* 22:366–369, 1972.
32. Ludvigsson J: Propranolol used in prophylaxis of migraine in children. *Neurol Scand* 50:109–115, 1974.
33. Vardi Y, Robey IM, Streifler M, Schwartz A, Lindner HR, Zor U: Migraine attacks: Alleviation by an inhibitor of prostaglandin synthesis and action. *Neurology* 26:447–450, 1976.
34. Kallanranta T, Hukkarainen H, Hokkanen E, Tuovinen T: Clonidine in migraine prophylaxis. *Headache* 17:169–172, 1977.
35. Keppel G: *Designs and Analysis: A Researcher's Handbook*. Englewood Cliffs, New Jersey, Prentice-Hall, 1973.

Chapter 10
A Study of Physicians' Attitude on Biofeedback

MAXINE L. WEINMAN, D. P.H.
ROY J. MATHEW, M.D.
JAMES L. CLAGHORN, M.D.

The widespread interest in clinical and research applications of biofeedback has been reflected in the establishment of two national biofeedback societies (Biofeedback Society of America and American Society of Biofeedback Clinicians) and numerous state societies, as well as two journals (*Biofeedback and Self-Regulation* and the *American Journal of Clinical Biofeedback*). The Task Force Report of the Biofeedback Society of America has recommended the use of biofeedback in six major areas: vascular headache [1], muscle-contraction headache [2], vasoconstrictive disorders (i.e., primary Raynaud's disease) [3], psychosociological disorders [4], gastrointestinal disorders [5], and physical medicine and rehabilitation [6]. Additionally, the proliferation of books on the subject written for the lay public has enhanced the appeal of biofeedback.

Many biofeedback issues are unresolved or controversial. Some insurance companies provide coverage for biofeedback therapy as part of a routine professional visit, some cover it only as a psychiatric service, while others may limit the eligibility of service providers or only reimburse policy holders for specific conditions. A related issue concerns the medical community's acceptance of biofeedback as a treatment modality, specifically for use recommended by the Biofeedback Society of America.

The purpose of our study was to survey attitudes and knowledge about biofeedback among physicians in the Harris County Medical Society. To detect patterns of response and avoid bias, the sample was stratified according to the proportional representation of specialties in the total population. Based on this stratification, questionnaires were mailed to a random sample of members of the Harris County Medical Society.

METHODS

A 10-percent proportionate sample of Harris County physicians was desired for the study. Certain physician specialties were not included in the research because they lacked relevancy to the subject matter—for example, anesthesiology, emergency medicine, and general preventive medicine. In 1978, 4,175 physicians were listed in the Harris County Medical Society roster, and 3,373 were eligible for the study. To achieve a 10-percent response, questionnaires were mailed to 1,181 physicians, a 35-percent random sample that was stratified according to proportional representation by specialty. The sampling by specialty was based on 19 categories; certain specialties were combined when individual numbers were small or when groupings were appropriate.

All responses to the questionnaire were coded by a specialty number to guarantee anonymity. The return was 465 questionnaires, or 38.6 percent of the sample, and 13.5 percent of the population total. The specialists in the total population, their proportion to the total population, their proportionate number in the survey sample and the response rate by specialty are presented in Table 1.

RESULTS

Knowledge of Biofeedback

The first question we asked the physicians concerned their overall knowledge about biofeedback. A scale from 1 to 5 was used, with 1 representing no knowledge and 5 being very knowledgeable. The overall response is presented in Table 2. Sixty-two percent of the respondents checked category 1 or 2, indicating relatively little knowledge, while 11.6 percent were in the most knowledgeable categories, 4 and 5. Twenty-three percent checked the middle category 3.

Examining these responses by specialty of physicians showed that neurologists, psychiatrists, and allergists had the majority of their re-

Table 1

Sample Frame and Response Rate of Harris County Physicians in Attitudinal Study on Biofeedback

Specialty	No. in Total Population (n = 3373)	Percentage of Total Population (n = 3373)	Proportionate No. in Survey Sample (n = 1181)	Response Rate by Specialty (percentage)
Aerospace medicine	24	0.71	8	25
Allergy	40	1.18	14	35.71
Cardiovascular disease	115	3.40	41	31.70
Dermatology	51	1.51	18	22.22
Endocrinology	51	1.51	18	50
Gastroenterology	36	1.07	13	76.92
General practice	522	15.47	183	36.06
Internal medicine	527	15.62	184	39.13
Neoplastic disease	39	1.15	14	21.42
Neurology	73	2.16	26	38.46
Obstetrics and gynecology	348	10.31	122	35.24
Occupational/physical medicine	86	2.55	30	46.66
Oncology	27	0.80	9	55.55
Ophthalmology	111	3.29	39	28.20
Otorhinolaryngology	75	2.22	26	34.61
Pediatrics	247	7.32	86	56.97
Psychiatry	275	8.15	96	48.95
Pulmonary disease	51	1.51	18	22.22
Surgery	675	20.01	236	33.89

Table 2

Physician Response to Biofeedback Questionnaire

"How Knowledgeable Are You About Biofeedback?"

Not At All 1		2		3		4		Very 5		No Response 6	
%	n	%	n	%	n	%	n	%	n	%	n
33.8	(154)	28.7	(131)	23.9	(109)	9.6	(44)	2.0	(9)	2.0	(9)

"Do You Use Biofeedback in Your Practice?"

Yes		No		No Response	
%	n	%	n	%	n
7.7	(35)	86.2	(393)	6.1	(28)

"Do You Refer Patients for Biofeedback?"

Yes		No		No Response	
%	n	%	n	%	n
21.7	(99)	72.1	(329)	6.1	(28)

"Do You Support Insurance Coverage for Biofeedback Treatment?"

Yes		No		Undecided		No Response	
%	n	%	n	%	n	%	n
27.6	(126)	16.9	(77)	47.1	(215)	8.3	(38)

sponses in categories 3 through 5. At the other extreme, 11 groups checked category 1 more frequently than any other: aerospace medicine, general practice, internal medicine, obstetrics and gynecology, neoplastic disease, oncology, occupational/physical medicine, ophthalmology, otorhinolaryngology, pediatrics, and surgery.

The Use of Biofeedback

The second questionnaire concerned the actual use of biofeedback in the physicians' practice. As shown in Table 2, 86.2 percent of the physicians did not use biofeedback. Of the 7.7 percent who responded "yes," eight of the 35 users were psychiatrists, seven were surgeons, five were occupational/physical medicine specialists and four were general practitioners. The rest were composed of internists (3), ophthalmologists (2), neurologists (2), obstetricians (2), with one endocrinologist and one otorhinolaryngologist.

Referral of Patients

The third question addressed the physicians' willingness to refer patients for biofeedback treatment. As seen in Table 2, 21.7 percent responded "yes." Specialty responses showed that psychiatrists, neurologists, and pulmonary disease specialists were the only majority "yes" responders. The "yes" response was generally represented across the various specialties, with the exception of aerospace medicine, cardiovascular disease, neoplastic disease, and oncology.

Insurance Coverage

The fourth item canvassed attitudes concerning health insurance coverage for biofeedback. As seen in Table 2, the largest response category was "undecided" (47.1 percent). Twenty-seven percent responded "yes," with dermatologists, psychiatrists, and neurologists having their majority response in this category. The "no" response (16.9 percent) did not receive any specialty majority.

Specific Application of Biofeedback

The next series of questions dealt specifically with indications for the use of biofeedback in the treatment of nine disorders. Physicians were asked to check either "primary" or "adjunct treatment" or "not indicated" for each disorder; "don't know/no opinion" and "not sure" categories were also created. The physicians' responses are presented in Table 3.

Table 3

Physician Attitude on Biofeedback as a Treatment for Selected Disorders

Disease	Primary Treatment		Adjunct Treatment		Not Indicated		Don't Know/ No Opinion		Not Sure	
	%	n	%	n	%	n	%	n	%	n
Migraine headaches	5.7	(26)	48.5	(221)	7.9	(36)	34.4	(157)	3.5	(16)
Muscle-contraction headaches	18.4	(84)	40.6	(185)	4.8	(22)	33.6	(153)	2.6	(12)
Raynaud's disease (idiopathic)	3.1	(14)	23.2	(106)	26.1	(119)	41.0	(187)	6.6	(30)
Fecal incontinence	4.2	(19)	22.4	(102)	23.2	(106)	42.3	(193)	7.9	(36)
Neuromuscular rehabilitation	5.0	(23)	38.2	(174)	11.6	(53)	39.9	(182)	5.3	(24)
Epilepsy	0.4	(2)	16.7	(76)	35.1	(160)	42.3	(193)	5.5	(25)
Relaxation training for anxiety and tension	25.9	(118)	35.5	(162)	3.9	(18)	32.5	(148)	2.2	(10)
Pain management	6.6	(30)	51.1	(233)	5.7	(26)	32.9	(150)	3.7	(17)
Essential hypertension	1.8	(8)	42.3	(193)	14.9	(68)	37.1	(169)	3.9	(18)

n = 456

Overall, the "primary treatment" response and the "not indicated" categories did not receive a majority response for any of the named disorders. "Adjunct treatment" was selected more frequently than any other response for migraine (49 percent), muscle-contraction headache (41 percent), relaxation training for anxiety and tension (36 percent), pain management (51 percent), and essential hypertension (42 percent). The "don't know/no opinion" category was selected most frequently for Raynaud's disease (idiopathic) (41 percent) and fecal incontinence (42 percent). Consistently, between 33 percent and 43 percent of all responses were in the "don't know" category.

Analysis of Biofeedback Use by Physician Specialty

Migraine headache

No specialty group selected "primary treatment" or "not indicated" for the majority response for migraine headache. "Adjunct treatment," the largest response category for migraine, was selected by all specialty groups except aerospace medicine and pulmonary disease. Twelve specialists chose "adjunct treatment" for the majority response. They were allergists, pulmonary disease specialists, dermatologists, psychiatrists, gastroenterologists, oncologists, internists, general practitioners, occupational medicine specialists, obstetricians/gynecologists, pediatricians, and endocrinologists. Neurologists had no majority preference, with 30 percent choosing the "adjunct treatment" category and 30 percent the "not indicated" category.

Muscle-contraction headache

The "primary treatment" category received the majority response from dermatologists and endocrinologists for muscle-contraction headaches. "Adjunct treatment," the largest response category, was selected by all specialty groups except aerospace medicine and neoplastic disease. Eight specialists chose "adjunct treatment" for the majority response. They were: allergists, psychiatrists, neurologists, occupational medicine, pulmonary disease, internists, general practitioners, and gastroenterologists. The "not indicated" category did not receive a majority response from any specialty.

Raynaud's disease

For Raynaud's disease (idiopathic), "primary treatment" did not receive a majority from any specialty. The largest overall response category was "don't know," the majority response from 14 specialty groups. The "not indicated" category showed representation from all groups except aerospace medicine, cardiovascular disease, and dermatology. Two groups, gastroenterologists and neurologists, had the majority response in this category. The "adjunct treatment" response was selected by all specialties except areospace medicine, allergy, neoplastic disease, and otorhinolaryngology. A majority of dermatologists and psychiatrists chose the "adjunct treatment" category.

Fecal incontinence

"Primary treatment" for fecal incontinence did not receive any specialist majority. The largest overall response was "don't know," the majority response from 14 specialty groups. The "not indicated" category was chosen by all groups except aerospace medicine, endocrinology, and oncology. A majority of neurologists, gastroenterologists and psychiatrists felt that biofeedback was not indicated in treatment of fecal incontinence. "Adjunct treatment" was picked by all specialties except aerospace medicine, neoplastic disease, oncology, and otorhinolaryngology. Allergists and dermatologists provided the majority response in this category.

Neuromuscular rehabilitation

No group selected "primary treatment" or "not indicated" as a majority response for biofeedback for neuromuscular rehabilitation. The largest overall response was "don't know," representing the majority response from nine specialties. "Adjunct treatment" was chosen by all groups, with the exception of aerospace medicine. Six specialists selected "adjunct treatment" as a majority response. They were dermatologists, psychiatrists, occupational-medicine specialists, neurologists, internists, and gastroenterologists.

Epilepsy

For epilepsy, the "primary treatment" response did not receive any specialist majority. "Adjunct treatment" was the majority response from dermatologists and psychiatrists. The largest overall response was "don't know," representing the majority response from 12 specialties. The "not indicated" category was selected by all specialties except aerospace medicine and dermatology. Neurologists, gastroenterologists, oncologists, and internists had the majority of their responses in this category.

Relaxation training for anxiety and tension

The "primary treatment" category for relaxation training for anxiety and tension received a majority response from oncologists. "Adjunct treatment" was the largest response category, selected by all groups except aerospace medicine, neoplastic disease, and oncology. Seven groups selected "adjunct treatment" as a majority response. They were allergists, dermatologists, gastroenterologists, internists, neurologists, psychiatrists, and pulmonary disease specialists. The "not indicated" category received no specialist majority.

Pain management

For pain management, the "primary treatment" and the "not indicated" category received no specialist majorities. "Adjunct treatment," the largest response category, was represented by all specialties, with the exception of aerospace medicine. Eleven groups selected "adjunct treatment" for a majority response. They were dermatologists, endocrinologists, gastroenterologists, general practitioners, internists, obstetricians/gynecologists, neurologists, occupational medicine specialists, pediatricians, psychiatrists, and pulmonary disease specialists. Surgeons were equally split between "adjunct treatment" and "don't know."

Essential hypertension

For the last disorder, essential hypertension, the "primary treatment" and the "not indicated" categories received no specialty majorities. "Adjunct treatment," the largest response category, was chosen by all groups except aerospace medicine. Nine groups selected "adjunct treatment" as a majority response. They were dermatologists, endocrinologists, general practitioners, internists, neurologists, oncologists, pediatricians, psychiatrists, and pulmonary disease specialists.

Analysis of Knowledge of Biofeedback

In general, physicians' responses regarding therapeutic interventions with biofeedback fell in the "adjunct treatment" and "don't know" categories. Analyses were conducted to ascertain whether the physicians' knowledge of biofeedback was related to their treatment choices.

Analysis was performed by comparing those physicians who were most knowledgeable about biofeedback, categories 3 to 5, with those who had little or no knowledge, categories 1 and 2 (Question 1). This comparison was carried out via the chi-square list of association for the responses to the nine specified disorders.

Migraine headache

For migraine headache, the most knowledgeable physicians selected "adjunct treatment" most frequently (65 percent), while the least knowledgeable selected "don't know" (48 percent). Only 10 percent of the most knowledgeable selected the "don't know" category for migraine headache, while 39 percent of the least knowledgeable selected "adjunct treatment" ($\chi^2 = 74.2$, $df = 4$; $p < .0001$).

Muscle-contraction headaches

For muscle contraction headaches, the most knowledgeable physicians selected "adjunct treatment" most frequently (58 percent), while the least knowledgeable selected "don't know" (48 percent). Nine percent of the most knowledgeable selected the "don't know" category for muscle-contraction headaches, while 31 percent of the least knowledgeable selected "adjunct treatment" ($\chi^2 = 74.53$, $df = 4$; $p < .0001$).

Raynaud's disease

Physicians' responses to Raynaud's disease showed that the most knowledgeable chose "adjunct treatment" most frequently (38 percent), followed closely by "not indicated" (30 percent). The least knowledgeable physicians selected the "don't know" category most frequently (53 percent), followed by "not indicated" (22 percent). Twenty percent of the most knowledgeable selected "don't know," while 15 percent of the least knowledgeable selected "adjunct treatment" ($\chi^2 = 61.25$, $df = 4$; $p < .001$).

Fecal incontinence

For fecal incontinence, the most knowledgeable physicians were divided between "adjunct treatment" (29 percent) and "not indicated" (30 percent) while the least knowledgeable selected "don't know" (51.2 percent). "Adjunct treatment" and "not indicated" received 18.6 percent and 18.9 percent respectively of the least knowledgeable physicians' responses ($\chi^2 = 25.73$, $df = 4$; $p < .0001$).

Neuromuscular rehabilitation

The most knowledgeable physicians chose "adjunct treatment" (54 percent) for neuromuscular rehabilitation, while those who were least knowledgeable selected "don't know" (52 percent). Twenty percent of the most knowledgeable selected "don't know," while 28 percent of the least knowledgeable selected "adjunct treatment" ($\chi^2 = 56.47$, $df = 4$; $p < .0001$).

Epilepsy

For epilepsy, the most frequent response from the most knowledgeable physicians was "not indicated" (45 percent), while the least knowledgeable selected "don't know" (53 percent). Twenty-five percent of the most knowledgeable selected the "don't know" category for epilepsy, while 29 percent of the least knowledgeable selected "not indicated" ($\chi^2 = 39.58, df = 4; p < .0001$).

Relaxation training for anxiety and tension

For relaxation training for anxiety and tension, the most frequent response from the most knowledgeable physicians was "adjunct treatment" (52 percent), while that of the least knowledgeable was "don't know" for relaxation training, and 26 percent of the least knowledgeable selected "adjunct treatment" ($\chi^2 = 86.21, df = 4; p < .0001$).

Pain management

The most knowledgeable physicians opted for biofeedback as an "adjunct treatment" in pain management (72 percent). The least knowledgeable selected "don't know" as their most frequent response (47 percent). Eight percent of the most knowledgeable selected "don't know" for pain management, while 39 percent of the least knowledgeable selected "adjunct treatment" ($\chi^2 = 74.89, df = 4; p < .0001$).

Essential hypertension

For essential hypertension, the most knowledgeable physicians chose "adjunct treatment" (60 percent), while the least knowledgeable selected "don't know" as their most frequent response (50 percent). Fifteen percent of the most knowledgeable selected "don't know," while 32 percent of the least knowledgeable selected "adjunct treatment" ($\chi^2 = 53.17, df = 4; p < .0001$).

The majority of responses by physicians with knowledge of biofeedback were in specific treatment categories, while those with little or no knowledge, however, had a much higher response to specific treatment categories than the physicians who were most knowledgeable had to the "don't know" category. A possible explanation is that although physicians are not knowledgeable about biofeedback, they respond positively to its use as an "adjunct treatment" for some disorders and negatively to its use for others.

SUMMARY

The results of this study indicated that the majority of physicians surveyed had little or no knowledge of biofeedback, did not use biofeedback in their practice, and were undecided about insurance coverage.

About one-quarter of all physicians referred patients for biofeedback treatment.

Regarding the use of biofeedback for specific disorders, the most frequent response was either "adjunct treatment" or "don't know/no opinion." The "primary treatment" category or "not indicated" categories received no majority response for any disorder.

Responses by physician specialty revealed that psychiatrists and neurologists were the most knowledgeable about biofeedback, with more psychiatrists referring patients and supporting insurance coverage than any other group.

Majority responses by specialty to the use of biofeedback as a treatment for specific disorders were difficult to interpret because of the large percentage of "don't knows." However, for those disorders for which "adjunct treatment" or "not indicated" received a high percentage of responses, most specialties were represented. Psychiatrists consistently dominated the majority response across all groups in the "adjunct treatment" category for specific disorders. The only exception was for fecal incontinence in which the "not indicated" category received the majority response.

These findings suggest that biofeedback, like other types of behavioral therapies, is supported as an "adjunct treatment" for some psychosomatic disorders. While it is too early to ascertain the role of biofeedback in the mainstream of medical treatment, its acceptance by the medical field will have an impact on its regulation. For conditions amenable to treatment, it is better for physicians to refer their patients to qualified biofeedback therapists rather than allowing the choice of therapists to be based on information from the mass media. For this reason, studies of community acceptance of biofeedback are important for physicians and biofeedback therapists. The results of this survey magnified the need for more information on the use of behavioral therapies by physicians; in their responses to this questionnaire many participants expressed their interest in learning more about biofeedback.

REFERENCES

1. Diamond S, Diamond-Falk J, DeVeno T: Biofeedback in the treatment of vascular headache. *Biofeedback and Self-Regulation* 3(4):385–408, 1978.
2. Fernando CK, Basmajian JV: Biofeedback in physical medicine and rehabilitation. *Biofeedback and Self-Regulation* 3(4): 435–455, 1978.
3. Fotopoulos SS, Sunderland WP: Biofeedback in the treatment of psychophysiologic disorders. *Biofeedback and Self-Regulation* 3(4):331–362, 1978.

4. Miller NE: Biofeedback and visceral learning. *Ann Review Psychol* 29:373–404, 1978.
5. Taub E, Stroebel CF: Biofeedback in the treatment of vasoconstrictive syndromes. *Biofeedback and Self-Regulation* 3(4):363–374, 1978.
6. Whitehead WE: Biofeedback in the treatment of gastrointestinal disorders. *Biofeedback and Self-Regulation* 3(4):375–384, 1978.

Index

Abortive treatment, for migraine, 33–34
Acetaminophen, 33
Acetazolamide (Diamox), 23
Acetylcholine, 79
Acetylsalicylic acid, 18
  See also Aspirin
Adaptation-relaxation reflex, 119
Adenosine triphosphate, 79
Age, as factor in biofeedback therapy, 58
Alpha enhancement, 129
Alpha feedback, and vascular headache, 52–53
Amaurosis fugax, 11
Amaurosis fugax vs. ophthalmic migraine, 11
American Journal of Clinical Biofeedback, 153
American Society of Biofeedback Clinicians, 153
Amitriptyline, 32
Amyl nitrite, 78
Analgesic units, 99
Anger, as factor in migraine, 129
Antidepressants, in treatment of migraine, 31–32
Antihypertensive drugs, in treatment of migraine, 27–29
Antiserotonergic drugs, in treatment of migraine, 29–31
Anxiety, 129, 130
  and monamine oxidase activity, 135
Arnold-Chiari malformation, 21
Arousal, as physiological basis of emotions, 55, 129

Arteriography, 23
Arteriosclerosis, 128
Arteriovenous malformation of the brain, clinical signs of, 16
Aspirin, 32–33
  See also Acetylsalicylic acid
Assertive therapy, 46–47
Autogenic biofeedback hand temperature control, 43
  with electromyographic and temperature feedback, 50–51
Autogenic feedback training, 38–39, 47, 80–81, 141
Autogenic relaxation phrases, 40, 105, 106, 129
Autogenic training and thermal biofeedback, results of treatment by, 148
Autonomic nervous system training, questions concerning, 128

Barratt Impulsiveness Scales, 42
Basilar artery migraine (Bickerstaff), 3, 4, 5, 9, 12–13
Basophil cell heparin, and migraine, 71–72
Bellergal, 30
Benign intracranial hypertension, 22–23
Biochemical mechanisms in migraine, 68–72
Biochemical pathways of platelet aggregation, 69
Biofeedback, 37, 92–121
  criticisms of, 92–93
  four possible outcomes of, 102–103
  future research goals, 59–60

increase in degree of control following, 128
insurance companies' policies toward, 153
medical community's attitude toward, 154–164
precautions and contraindications, 56–58
and psychotherapeutic variables, 106–107
and relaxation, 105
results of research in, 54–56
review of, 38–54
therapeutic efficacy of, 128
training, 58–59, 96–97, 128
volitional control over autonomic functions as basis of, 127
Biofeedback, attitudinal study on, 153–154, 155, 156, 163–164
health insurance coverage for, 157
knowledge of, 154, 157, 161–163
referral of patients, 157
specific application of, 157, 158, 159–160
use of, 157
Biofeedback and Self-Regulation, 153
Biofeedback Society of America, 153
Bradykinin, 79
Brain tumor headache, 16–18
Bromocryptine, 31

CAT scan of brain in acute obstructive hydrocephalus, 22
CAT scan of brain showing low-density area in parietal region, 12
Catecholamine, and migraine, 4, 129–130
effect of relaxation on levels of, 130–135
Cephalic vasoconstriction, *see* Vasoconstriction of the extracranial artery
Cephalic vasomotor response feedback (CVMR), 45, 147
Children, and biofeedback, 58
Classic migraine, 3, 4, 9, 11, 95
cerebral blood flow (CBF) changes in, 67
differentiated from arteriovenous malformation headache, 16, 17
plasma serotonin changes in, 68

Clinical summary of 9 cases of basilar artery migraine, 13
Clonidine (Catapres), 3, 5, 6
in treatment of migraine, 29
Cluster headache, 4, 5
Cognitive set, as therapeutic variable, 107
Combined desensitization, 46
Common migraine, 4, 5, 95
and combined-modality biofeedback training, 52
Complicated migraine, 4
classified, 9–10
definition of, 9
differentiated from transient ischemic attacks, 24
general characteristics of, 10
ocular complications of, 10–11
Corticosteroids, 23
CO_2 inhalation, cerebral vasodilator response to 3, 4, 5, 7
Cultivated low arousal, 106
Curare, 128
Cyproheptadine, 29–30

Dandy-Walker syndrome, 21
Deep muscle relaxation therapy, 45, 46
vs. biofeedback for treatment of migraine, 47
and thermal feedback, 48
Deficient nociception, as cause of migraine, 73
Dexamethasone, 34
Differential diagnosis of migraine, 13, 14–15
Digital vasodilation, and biofeedback, 46
Dihydroergotamine, 34
Dihydroergotoxine (Hydergine), 5, 6
Dipyridamol, 32–33
Drug dependency, and biofeedback training, 58

Effects of placebo on migraine headache, 149
Emotional factors, in personality of migraine patient, 57
Enhanced awareness, as component in migraine treatment, 106
Epilepsy, 160, 162–163

INDEX

Epinephrine, 7, 78
  and stress, 129, 130
Ergotamine tartrate, 30, 33–34, 69, 78
  contraindications for, 34
Essential hypertension, 161, 163
Estrogen, and migraine, 70–71

Fecal incontinence, 160, 162, 164
Fick principle, 1
Free fatty acids (FFA), 68, 69, 130
Frontalis EMG feedback, 45, 46, 85–86, 129, 142
  and thermal feedback, 47–50
Furosemide (Lasix), 23

Gastrointestinal disorders, 153
Glycerol, 23
Gray matter atrophy, 1

Hand temperature control, 41–44, 83
Hand warming, therapeutic efficacy of, 54–55, 85–86, 128
  See also Skin temperature control
Headache, classification of conditions that cause, 14–15
Headache associated with brain tumor, 16–18
Hemicrania, 4
Hemiparetic migraine, 12
Hemiplegic migraine, 9, 11–12
Hemispheric cerebral blood flow and headache variables, correlations between, 115
Histamine, 73, 79
Hydrocephalus, 17
Hypercapnia, 4, 7
Hypnosis, 142
  as factor in biofeedback, 42–43
  vs. temperature biofeedback, 53–54
Hypoglycemia, 130
Hypothalamus, role of, in migraine, 79, 80

Increased intracranial pressure, and headache, 20
  benign intracranial hypertension, 22–23
  obstruction of cerebrospinal fluid pathways, 20–22

Intracerebral circulation, and temperature biofeedback, 43–44
Intracerebral hematoma, and headache, 20
Intracranial aneurysms, and headache, 15
  ruptured, 16
Intracranial and extracranial vasodilation during migraine, 128
Intracranial pressure, increase in, 20–22
Intracranial vasoconstriction, and onset of migraine, 51, 67, 78, 128
Iron-deficiency anemia, 130
Ischemia, and migraine, 67
Ischemic cerebrovascular disease, and headache, 23–24
Isometheptene (Midrin), 5, 34
Isoproterenol (Isuprel), 5, 6

Jacobson's relaxation technique, 129, 142
Juvenile migraine, 13

Mean percentage of change in headache variables after feedback training, 100
Meditation, and migraine, 80, 86, 105, 127, 142
  See also Relaxation procedures
Meningitis, 18, 21
Menstrual migraine, and estrogen, 70
Meta-analysis, 141, 148
  results of, 149–150
Methysergide, 30
Migraine, 91, 95, 103–104, 159, 161–162
  biochemical mechanisms in, 68–72
  as circulatory disturbance, 79
  differential diagnosis of, 13–25
  hemodynamics in, 115–116
  historical perspective of, 78–80
  as multisystemic disorder, 74
  pain mechanisms in, 72–74
  pathogenesis of, 71, 72, 73
  treatment of, with various forms of relaxation, 141–150
Migraine pain mechanism, two theories of, 72–74
Migraine personality, 57
Monoamine oxidase (MAO), 70, 80, 130
  effect of relaxation on levels of, 130–135
Muscle contraction headache, 4, 5, 95, 153, 159, 162

INDEX

Muscle tension, in vascular headache, 51

Neurogenic theory of migraine headache (Wolff), 4, 38
Neurologists, attitude of, toward biofeedback, 164
Neuromuscular rehabilitation, 160, 162
Norepinephrine, 7, 78
  and stress, 129

Ocular paralysis, 15
Ophthalmic migraine, 11
Ophthalmoplegic migraine, 10
Otitic hydrocephalus, 22–23

Pain management, 161, 163
Pain mechanisms of migraine, 72–74
Papilledema, 21, 22
Parietal arteriovenous malformation, 17
Passive concentration, to induce physiological changes, 38
Patient undergoing Xe inhalation measurement of rCBF, 2
Peripheral vasoconstriction, and migraine, 51, 67
Phenelzine, 31
Phenylethylamine, 69, 70
Physical medicine and rehabilitation, 153
Pitozifen (Sandomigran), 30–31
Placebo, 104, 147
  effects of, on migraine headache, 149
Platelet inhibitors, in treatment of migraine, 32–33
Pneumoencephalography, 23
Polygraph, 2
Polymyalgia rheumatica syndrome, and headache, 24–25
Premenstrual tension, 130
Propranolol (Inderal), 5, 6, 11
  in treatment of migraine, 28–29
Prostaglandins (PG), 69
Pseudotumor cerebri, 22–23
Psychiatrists, attitude of, toward biofeedback, 164
Psychological factors, and migraine patient, 57
Psychophysiological feedback, 82
Psychophysiology of emotional states, 106
Psychosociological disorders, 153

Psychosomatic self-regulation, 80, 87
  and autogenic feedback training, 81, 83–85
  biofeedback as adjunct treatment, 164
  integration into medical therapies, 87
  in migraine treatment, 81–86
  rationale for, 80–81

Raynaud's disease, 128, 153, 159–160, 162
Regional cerebral blood flow (rCBF), 1–2, 5
  application to migraine research, 3–7, 78, 97
  in normal vs. migraine patients, 112–113
  skin temperature regulation and change in, 110–115
  values of, 3, 4
Regional cerebral blood flow and skin temperature self-regulation, correlations between, 114
Relative potency scale, 99
Relaxation training, 52, 80, 98, 110, 141–147, 160–161, 163
  biochemical rationale for, 118
  effect on monoamine oxidase, 135
  key role of, 104–105, 127, 129
  rationale for, 141
  and skin temperature training, 105–106
  vs. thermal biofeedback, 147–150
  See also Meditation
Relaxation training to treat migraine headache, summary of studies using, 144–146
REM sleep, 130
Ruptured intracranial aneurysms, and headache, 16

Scotoma, 10
  scintillating, 11
Self-induced hypnotic relaxation, and headache, 52–53, 98, 129
Self-report of headache data, 107–108
Serotonin, 68, 69, 78
  in pain mechanism of migraine, 72–73, 130
Serotonin theory of migraine, 135
Skin conductance, 129

Skin temperature control, in migraine, 92–99, 120–121, 129
  absolute vs. temperature change, 108–109
  vs. cephalic vasoconstriction, 119–120
  hand-warming vs. hand-cooling, 101–102, 111–112
  and headache variables, 102
  relationship between hand trained and rCBF, 115
  and relaxation, 105–106
  relevance of, 128–129
  and stage of headache, 118
  symptomatic vs. prophylactic application of, 109–110
  See also Temperature biofeedback
Skin temperature self-regulation and headache data, correlation between, 103
Sleep disturbance, 58
Sodium iodide, 1
State anxiety, 131
State-Trait Anxiety Inventory, 42, 130, 131
Stress, and migraine, 51, 82, 106, 110, 129, 135
Subarachnoid hemorrhage, and headache, 15–16
Subdural hematoma, and headache, 19–20
Sulfinpyrazone, 32–33
Summary of results of testing with isometheptene, 6
Sympathetic arousal, 141
Sympathetic outflow theory, 55
Sympathetic tone, 129

Target training, 42
Task Force Report (Biofeedback Society of America), recommendations of, 153
Temperature biofeedback, 43–44, 54–56, 141
  and autogenic training, 141, 150
  and electromyographic feedback, 48–50, 86, 98
  hypothesized mechanisms of, 116–118
  and psychotherapy as treatment, 51–52
  and relaxation, 150
  See also Skin temperature control
Temporal arteritis, and headache, 24–25
Thermal feedback, see Temperature biofeedback
Thermal feedback, results of treatment by, 148
Thermal training, and migraine, 80, 85–86, 87
  See also Skin temperature control
Trait anxiety, 131
Transcendental meditation, 129
  See also Meditation
Treatment of migraine, 27
  preventive, 27–33
  symptomatic, 33–34
Tic douloureux, 18
Tolossa-Hunt syndrome, and headache, 25
Transient ischemic attacks (TIA), with headache, 23–24
Tumors, and headache, 18–19
Tyramine, as cause of headaches, 57, 69, 130

Vascular headache, 91, 153
  etiology of, 57
  types of, 37
Vasoconstriction of the extracranial artery, and biofeedback, 44–45, 119–120, 153
Venipuncture, 132

Xenon (Xe) inhalation method, 1–2, 78, 97

Yoga, see Meditation